The Power of Flowers

Healing Body and Soul
Through the Art and Mysticism of Nature

First Edition

Library of Congress Cataloging-in-Publication Data

Lerner, Isha, 1954-

Power of Flowers: Healing Body and Soul Through the Art and Mysticism of Nature/Isha Lerner.

p. cm.

Includes bibliographical references.

ISBN 1-57281-257-5

1. Flowers—Therapeutic use. 2. Mysticism. 3. Healing.

4. Homeopathy—Materia medica and therapeutics. I. Title

RX615.F55.L47 2000

615.8'9—dc21

00 10 9 8 7 6 5 4 3 2 1

Printed in Canada

U.S. Games Systems, Inc.
179 Ludlow Street
Stamford, CT 06902 USA

The Power of Flowers

Healing Body and Soul
Through the Art and Mysticism of Nature

by Isha Lerner

Illustrations by Karen Forkish

U.S. GAMES
SYSTEMS, INC

Published by
U.S. GAMES SYSTEMS, INC.
Stamford, CT 06902 USA

Dedication

May the flowers bless my dear Sophie,
and all the children of the earth.

Acknowledgements

I wish to acknowledge the late Edward Bach for his sensitive
and untiring dedication to the study of nature and flower
essence therapy; Richard Katz and Patricia Kaminsky for their
contribution to flower essence research through The Flower
Essence Society; Tara McKinney for her wise editing and
inspiration; Gabrielle, Katya, and Sophie, my three daughters,
for being the "flowers of joy" in my own garden of life;
Karen Forkish for her fantastic illustrations and friendship; and
Stuart Kaplan of U.S. Games Systems, Inc., Elizabeth Kerkstra,
and Dana Duncan O'Kelly for their support in helping
this project blossom into the world.

—Isha Lerner

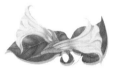

Dedication

To my daughter Madeleine Gagne,
with love and gratitude, now and always.

Acknowledgements

Heartfelt thanks to my family for their constant love and
support in this and all things. I would also like to note my deep
appreciation of Pamela Lehan-Siegel and Marc Siegel of the
Dance Theatre of Oregon, Shannon McDonald, Mark Allee, and
Madeleine for their patient modelling.

—Karen Forkish

Flower Reference

Table of Contents

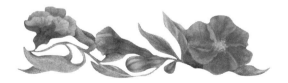

*Cover my Earth Mother four times
with many flowers.*

— A Zuni song

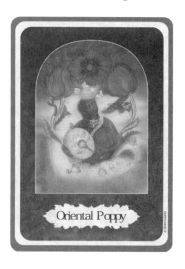

Oriental Poppy

The Power of Flowers

The love affair between the floral kingdom and humankind stretches back a very long way, perhaps to the first Neanderthal to pick a handful of posies for the purpose of brightening her cave. Over the centuries, careworn people everywhere have found that beautiful blossoms lift their spirits and touch their hearts in mysterious ways. Flowers have inspired countless legends and myths, associating them with various deities and nature spirits. During the Victorian era, an elaborate flower-based language became the mode of courtship and friendship, in that each flower included in a bouquet was understood to convey a particular message.

Flowers continue to enjoy almost universal appeal. Unfortunately we are losing touch with the legends and myths that echo the human heart's instinctive communion with the plant kingdom. *The Power Of Flowers*, illustrated by Karen Forkish, restores our awareness of these ancient associations. Isha Lerner's background in mythology and her knowledge of the spiritual underpinnings of plant life are richly evident in this work. For those of us who are uplifted and healed by myth, as well as by our connection to the feminine branch of the divine, this deck can serve as a delightful tool for reconnecting with the healing power of nature, in general, and with the plant kingdom, in particular.

The deck and book set can also be a valuable tool for choosing and working with the increasingly popular flower remedies made by such companies as Bach and The Flower Essence Society. Flower remedies, also known as essences, are a gentle healing tool of great beauty and hope, an alternative vibrational medicine akin to homeopathy. For well over a decade, I have incorporated these remedies into my astrological and counseling work. As a result, I have watched people release layer after layer of self-created obstacles; opening their hearts and souls to new life, much as flower buds open, little by little. It has become clear to me that people, even my grim-faced fellow New Yorkers (many of whom had never seen a flower grow), are deeply connected to the plants whose energies permeate the essences. Many of my clients who took flower essences had striking dreams, profound insights, and spontaneous bouts of forgiveness, all with life altering effects.

This form of subtle body healing can proceed without contact with plants and their overseer spirits, called devas, of course. Yet, the healing went so much further when the person worked consciously with these energies. I often showed my clients pictures of the flowers whose essences they were taking, and even this momentary contact was like a sunburst illuminating their faces. I also made certain they were conscious of the special properties of their remedies, so that these properties could be invoked with each dose. In addition, I found that affirmations and visualizations of the desired results seemed to sharpen the intent, causing the healing to proceed with greater speed, clarity and depth.

The stunning floral images in this card deck, along with the grace-filled explanations and meditations that accompany each flower, can take flower remedy work even further, acting in accordance with the essences to deepen their impact. If you love flowers, you will love working even more consciously with them through The Power of Flowers.

Donna Cunningham, MSW
Author of "Flower Remedies Handbook"
Portland, Oregon
Spring, 1997

The Power of Flowers

*The elders have asked that the morning after every
full moon at 10:00 a.m. that we gather and that
we go outside and we look to the Sun, to the flowers, and to the heart of the earth....In doing so we
bring more solar energy and flower wisdom to the
earth, because the next age is the Age of Flowers.
Flowers are our medicine for the next age.*

—Ven. Dhyana Ywahoo
Clan Chieftaness, Cherokee Nation

*P*lants—whether flowers, herbs, roots, or trees—have
been in the business of healing humanity for as long
as the two have co-existed on this planet. And, fortunately,
throughout recorded history, the special healing properties
of plants have been documented and made available to us
in various forms. Now, after many years of gestation, this
"Medicine of the Earth" is being offered in a most unusual,
yet practical, fashion, through The Power of Flowers deck
and accompanying book. This project, the culmination of all
that I have lived until now, explores the intricate mysteries
of plant healing from a number of perspectives, intertwin-
ing occult knowledge of flower essences, gardening,
astrology, tarot, alchemy, archetypal psychology, art, and
color therapy. I offer this fertile "Secret Garden" to you as a
prayer of hope to Mother Earth and all of Her inhabitants,
and for Her graceful survival into the New Millennium.

I first encountered what might be called "the feminine
soul of nature," or Natura, as a young woman living on the
Hawaiian Islands. One day as I sat on the shores of the Kauai

coast, amidst green ferns and red hibiscus flowers, a rush of violet light suddenly filtered across my vision. Within seconds, I was aware of intricate patterns of beautiful, translucent color surrounding the plants in my vicinity. These plant auras shimmered and glowed like stars and diamonds, enchanting me with their visual music. Other encounters with Nature's muse would follow, but the power of this first experience has never left me. It was a profound opening to the wonders of the natural world—a gift of spirit, for which I will always be grateful, and without which I could not have brought this project to fruition. In my mind, I heard the words "welcome home" sweetly whispered, and knew that I had been granted a rare invitation into the secret world of fairies and flowers. I also understood that the vague feeling of homesickness which had always haunted me—even in my happiest moments—was, in fact, a longing for this place, my true home.

Change can happen very quickly when one is ready, willing, and able to be transformed. My magical interlude with nature had set the wheels of change in motion. Within the hour, I had made the acquaintance of a woman on the beach who happened to be reading a book about the Findhorn Foundation, a global community founded in the 1960's in northern Scotland to promote spiritual harmony between human beings and the rest of the natural world. Though I had no knowledge of Findhorn at that time, I was drawn to the book like a fish to water. Noting my excitement, the woman impulsively gave me her copy of the book and I immediately read it from cover to cover.

Synchronicity is a guardian angel who guides us to the right place at the right time. Upon returning from my island backpacking trip, I met a new housemate, Christopher, who had just arrived from Findhorn, having spent several years there coordinating work in the community kitchen. Thanks to his connections and generous assistance, within two short weeks I had received a special invitation from Findhorn's co-founder Peter Caddy, and was on my way to Scotland as part of a group charged with readying the newly purchased Cluny Hill Hotel for conferences, guest programs, and community life. And, so it was at age twenty-three, that I was given the opportunity to begin my true life's work. The ensuing years spent toiling in Findhorn kitchens and gardens (1976 - 1980) were to establish the general direction of my adult life—a path from which I have not wavered. Immersed in the very soul of nature, I vowed that one day I would find a way to share the wonder of all that I had experienced there. With the completion of The Power of Flowers, I have fulfilled this vow.

I began this project with the intention of incorporating masculine and feminine archetypes equally into The Power of Flowers cards, in the interest of promoting a balance of these energies in the world at large. And, initially, as I surrendered to the well of inspiration from which the archetypes associated with these cards emerged, masculine and feminine archetypes presented themselves in more or less equal measure. However, as I surrendered further to the process, I began to see that underlying each of the masculine archetypes was an even deeper feminine one, quietly making her presence known to me. Along with this insight, arose an awareness that these feminine archetypes were to be the primary source of inspiration for this work.

This is not to suggest that masculine archetypes are without therapeutic value. However, while the masculine archetypes depicted in The Power of Flowers deck are powerful images designed to assist in healing the wounded aspects of the human community, in general, and of the masculine principle, in particular, they must be understood to exist within the context of an all encompassing feminine matrix. I have gradually come to see that the pattern of masculine archetypes arising out of more fundamental feminine ones is a profound expression of the natural way of things.

The implications of honoring the feminine principle in the form of Mother Nature are nothing short of revolutionary and enlightening. On this point, I am in agreement with those who argue that the survival of humankind, as well as the evolution of consciousness, itself, depends upon it. We find ourselves at a moment in time unlike any other, for as we approach the great challenge and opportunity of the Millennium, we are called to reconnect with the vital forces of planetary healing to an unprecedented degree. To accomplish a healing of the magnitude required of us, we must apply all of the resources at our disposal to the daunting task of reinventing myths and archetypes in a manner which truly balances masculine and feminine principles without distorting either in turn.

Clearly, we will not reclaim the wisdom of Natura through wishful thinking. Rather, we must actively engage with Her in the context of the greater cosmology. Holding the seeds of future manifestations, flowers are microcosmic mandalas of this Great Womb we call our universe. They function, if only we will let them, as a "rainbow bridge to enlightenment." Therefore, turning to flowers for help with the challenges now confronting our culture makes good sense. With their color, scent, sacred geometry, and form, flowers reflect the purity, joy, and beauty that is held within the human heart. We must learn to listen with our hearts to the teachings of the flowers in order to realign ourselves with them; thereby raising our vibratory rate to that of Divine Creativity.

The Power of Flowers deck contains thirty-two cards, each depicting a particular flower associated with a human archetype or myth. This association illustrates the profound interdependence of spiritual and temporal worlds. Flowers act as mirrors to the human realm, and in their purest meeting, aid in the process of "actualizing the divine" within each individual. As the crowning glory of nature, flowers, with their delicate yet vibrant essence, awaken us to the angelic realm, serving as an elixir to the human soul—a remedy for the maladies that plague the human spirit. As we journey through nature's garden gates, we yield to the mysteries of the divine feminine. Once inside these gates, Her flowers teach us the Earth's organic, alchemical movement toward perfection, revealing themselves as holographic reflections of the various archetypes living within the deepest recesses of humanity.

Flowers and The Power of Flowers cards which invoke their presence, offer themselves up for the privilege of helping each of us embrace our destiny as spiritual beings—to fully awaken our inherently wise and compassionate natures. In our quest for liberation into the world, rather than from the world, it seems fitting that we turn to the world, itself, the natural world, for assistance and inspiration. In this great experiment we call evolution, perhaps the collaboration between human beings and flower beings will prove most fruitful of all. Patiently blossoming in our hearts, the flowers are eager to assist in the reemergence of the divine feminine, for it is She who must lead the way to a new world order, a New Millennium—one in which masculine and feminine energies are truly understood, honored, and balanced.

Chapter 1

Natura

The Soul of Nature

*Astrologers, those who have studied the stars,
and herbalists, those who have studied the plants,
have ever been seeking those remedies which will
help us to keep our health and joy.*

— Edward Bach

My intention in this chapter is to bring forward the key components that enhance the healing properties of flowers and nature so that the reader may gain the greatest possible benefit from the Power of Flowers cards. The key components are: alchemy, flower essences, and art—as these traditions relate to one another. If the entire natural world, including the world of human beings, is engaged in the alchemical process of spiritual transmutation, then flowers—both in the form of essences and of artistic renderings—are perhaps its greatest ally.

Alchemy

The ancient art of alchemy is almost as old as civilization itself. At the esoteric level, Western alchemists, in their quest for spiritual perfection, developed a tradition of "cosmic magic." It can be traced as far back as the 4th century B.C.E. (Before the Common Era), extending deep into the mystery of Thoth, the Egyptian god of mathematics and science. It is interesting to note that in the Eastern world of approximately the same time period, Hindu, Buddhist, and Taoist yogis were engaged in highly esoteric, alchemical experimentation, as well. In the Hindu and Buddhist context, these secret practices are commonly known as tantra.

At a more mundane level, Western alchemical theory is based on the notion that the material world, despite its great diversity of form, can be reduced to a single, primary substance. This substance, known as prima materia, or primal, chaotic matter, ultimately consists of four basic elements: air, fire, water, and earth. It was further believed that certain transmuting agents, themselves made up of these four basic elements, were capable of changing one material into another. In this context, alchemy was understood as the art of transmuting base materials into more refined materials through a process of freeing the original base materials from their "impurities." This notion became known as "the philosopher's stone"—the most recognized of all alchemical ideas. Perhaps Paraselsus described this alchemical movement toward purity and perfection best when he said:

> Nature...does not produce anything that is perfect in itself. Humanity must bring things to perfection. The work of bringing things to perfection is called "Alchemy" and he is an alchemist who carries what nature grows for the use of humanity to its destined end.

Alchemists of ancient times were not yet burdened by the artificial distinction between science and the occult. In this sense, they were at a decided advantage over modern day seekers of perfection. The observable world of nature and the invisible, unconscious world of the psyche were not yet dualistically set apart, allowing for a holistic approach to inner and outer realities. In a world of whole things, one was more apt to discover whole truths. The minds of antiquity were more fluid; imaginations more fertile, giving rise to fanciful visions and elaborate excursions into overlapping philosophical, psychological, and religious domains. Steeped in a profound and direct experience of the mystical union of matter and spirit, all material forms were recognized as ultimately changeable and transmutable.

The contribution made to both mystical and scientific enterprises by early alchemists cannot be overstated. They understood the elemental healing properties of various plants, flowers, and chemicals, and were, consequently, able to formulate many powerful elixirs and potions—including the herbal concoctions used in the Egyptian mummification process, as well as those used in African shamanic healing and visionary journeys. Ultimately, their greatest achievement was their exploration of the dark, mysterious, unconscious aspects of nature and humanity. Through this journey, the early alchemists managed a blend of the exotic, the scientific, the esoteric, and the mundane.

The imaginative quality of alchemical experimentation gave rise to a deep understanding of the nature of archetypes and their relationship to the material world. In the alchemical view, the archetypal realm takes precedence over the material in the sense that the former can be said to infuse the latter with divine order and meaning. As the higher vibratory patterns characteristic of archetypal energy become manifest within nature's myriad forms, they act as holographic seeds of radiant light, providing the sacred imprint for each newly-cast body, each living thing: the planets, stars, plants, trees, birds, animals, and human beings. The Hellenistic alchemist Hermes Trismegistus, known as the medieval Mercurius, referred to this archetypal design which lives within the body and soul of nature as "the Master Builder" or "Mara of Things."

Perhaps the most provocative alchemical symbol representing an archetypal pattern is that of the vessel. This symbol suggests a world in which form provides the container for the formless. Even the great canopy of stars and the umbrella of cosmic constellations seem held together by something bigger than themselves—a sacred container of infinite proportions. Pregnant with all possibilities, this vessel is a potent symbol of the mother matrix, the womb, gestation, the fertile inner recesses.

Beneath the surface of our daily lives, we are always asking the question, "Who am I, really, and where is my true home?" The answer to this question is so utterly obvious, so beautiful, so ordinary, and yet so profound, that, like the nose on our face, we have a hard time seeing it. Because of our own self-imposed limitations, the answer to this mystery can only be revealed little by little, as if a great veil were being lifted inch by inch, until the truth is completely exposed. Yet, we are destined to receive this knowledge.

The alchemical movement toward purity and perfection which is our birthright as spiritual/material beings, ushers us ever closer to the truth of who we really are and where we belong. Ancient alchemists believed that the natural world held the key to unlocking this mystery. Alchemical texts taught that in order to relate properly to nature, one must follow the "truth of imagination." This was not unlike the practice of meditation, where the seeker opens herself to channels of higher guidance and inspiration. Ideally, then, alchemists walked the gardens and forests of the Earth with astute concentration and attunement.

As the veil is lifted, the truth is revealed: we are each of us the High Priestess; our bodies Her temple. We were present at the birth of this universe, and beyond that, at the death of the one that came before. We heard the first sound vibration and the first spoken word. We birthed chaos into form and became known as the Empress Sophia, Mother of the World, whose love of wisdom opened the gates to the heart of wholeness. We are the Anima Christi, the feminine face of God. We are the Black Madonna, unafraid of dark, watery, womblike spaces. We are Tara, the first fully enlightened female Buddha, Goddess of the Lotus, also known, in the Chinese context, as QuanYin. We are Isis who holds alchemical secrets concerning the evolution and destiny of the human race.

According to Egyptian mythology, Isis was given her knowledge of the occult by a great angel, and instructed to keep it to herself, telling only her son Horus. Some of the information imparted to her has come down to us in the following passage:

Who is the sower and who is the harvester? One who sows barley will also harvest barley and one who sows wheat will also harvest wheat. Realize from that this is the whole creation and the whole process of coming into being, and know that a man is only able to produce a man, and a lion a lion, and a dog a dog, and if something happens contrary to nature (contrary to the law) then it is a miracle and cannot continue to exist, because nature enjoys nature, an nature impregnates nature, and nature overcomes nature... one must stay with existing nature and the matter one has in hand in order to prepare things. Just as I said before, wheat creates wheat, and a man begets a man, and thus also gold will harvest gold, like produces like. Now I have manifested the mystery to you.

The sentiments expressed in this paragraph are reminiscent of the alchemical insight encapsulated in the phrase "As above, so below," attributed to Hermes in The Emerald Tablets. We are not separate from the stars and the seeds, nor the heaven and the earth. Neither are we separate from the living essence which sustains and supports us, and is alive in every object. This is the spirit which overlights and animates the natural world.

The angel gives Isis knowledge, which she takes into herself and becomes. In this way, Isis is not apart from the mystery, nor is the mystery apart from her. Ultimately, Isis fills her vessel with the knowledge of inner, alchemical marriage or union. She begets a son, Horus, who embodies the knowledge, and is one with her. The Isis story runs parallel to the biblical story of Eve in the Garden of Eden, but with an entirely different interpretation. Whereas, the knowledge given Isis by the angel is considered a sacrament, furthering the cause of human evolution. Eve's act of eating the apple from the Tree of Knowledge has been interpreted as the source of Original Sin, or separation from God.

What alchemy teaches us is that occult knowledge has the potential to lead us toward our own perfection rather than away from it. The choice is always ours to make. What we do with the information we are given is up to us. We are all made in the image of The Divine. Likewise, nature is the Divine Mother, the vessel of life which contains our origins. Our bodies are but temporal imprints of this splendor, cast into form by a design of infinite possibilities and magnificence.

Flower Essences

Through the ages, shamans, priests and priestesses, medicine women and men, herbal alchemists, botanists, and holy people from all walks of life have sought a clearer understanding of the natural world around them. They have listened reverently to the voice of Nature, approaching Her as one approaches a beloved consort. In turn, through Her trees, flowers, seeds, leaves, fruits, and berries, She has offered the knowledge of healing and sustainability, revealing Herself fully only to those who will listen with heart and soul.

Our medicines of today have evolved from the study of herbology, botany, and biology. The healing properties of herbs have been identified through the centuries by studying their growth cycles, appearance, location, color, and movement. Homeopathy is yet another way in which plants are employed as healers. As with the teachings of Isis, we learn through homeopathy that like cures like, and nature overcomes nature. Human beings are readily cured, soothed, and enlightened by the medicinal magic of plants. The more we are in tune with the vibration of the soul of nature, the more She will impart Her gifts. There have been many pioneers in the field of alternative medicine who have listened intently enough to receive nature's teachings. For example, pictures from the early Renaissance era show herbalists and alchemists at work concocting elixirs, remedies, salves, and tinctures.

More recently, pioneering work in these fields has brought to our attention the healing properties of high vibrational healing modalities. The word vibration has become synonymous with energy, for we have learned that our bodies are fields of vibrating energy. Contained within each person's energetic field are at least seven major energy centers known as chakras. The relationship of these centers to physical and spiritual well-being has been studied by

Eastern teachers and religious adepts since antiquity. Fortunately, due to a resurgence of interest in esoteric matters, we are once again undertaking this kind of study. As we open in this way, it is imperative that we study the energetic fields and vibrational patterns of the rest of the natural world, as well, for we deny the wisdom of Mother Nature at our own peril.

One of the great names in the field of vibrational healing is Edward Bach, the founding father of the Bach Flower essences which he brought to the attention of the medical establishment in England in the 1930's. Dr. Bach was a sensitive and contemplative man who dedicated his life to humanity, tirelessly seeking ways by which to alleviate human suffering and bring joy to the human spirit. A medical doctor steeped in the integral field of homeopathy, Dr. Bach began to case study the healing effects of the flower's essence, which he had discovered while collecting dew drops from plants at dawn. Theorizing that such drops contained the energy pattern or signature of the plant from which it was derived, he further supposed that when ingested by human beings, the essence of the flower would match vibrational patterns stored within the genetic miasmas of the human body.

How fortunate for us that Dr. Bach was such an astute observer of the plant kingdom, for his theories proved correct. His thirty-eight remedies have aided humanity for over sixty years, paving the way for other, like-minded individuals to engage in similar efforts—creating new varieties of flower essences for the greater good. Flower essences were around before Dr. Bach's discoveries, however. It is conjectured by mystics and historians that they were widely in use in Atlantis and Lemuria, and, of course, in Egypt. Vibrational healing modalities, in general, are also not new. For example, the art of gem healing was and continues to be a common practice in the East. China has embraced flowers for their healing properties for centuries, and sound and color vibrations are thought to have played a very significant, therapeutic role in ancient Egypt.

The process by which a flower creates its own essence is nothing less than alchemical, for the four elements are readily used and vital in the process: earth sustains the seed and root system; air offers oxygen and wind helping to fertilize the plant; fire, in the form of sunlight, brings light and growth, drawing the plant toward the heavens; and water feeds the plant, expanding its properties in order that it may produce the juice or dew, the essence of the plant.

Since it is not feasible to generate enough flower essences for a growing population by collecting dew from the plants, a more efficient, though nonetheless alchemical, process has been developed. The system involves placing flower petals in a clear glass or crystal bowl of pure water which is then set in the Sun for a certain prescribed period of time so that the healing properties of the flower can be transferred from the flower to the water. The soul consciousness of the person collecting the essences is an important part of the equation, as is the placement of moon, stars, and planets. Once the essence or pattern of the flower is transferred to the water, the water is carefully collected in vials, preserved with alcohol or vinegar, and made available for use. If you are interested in making essences yourself, I recommend how-to manuals published by the flower essence companies listed in the Resource Directory at the back of the book.

Flower essences are elixirs or tinctures, not to be confused with aromatherapy, which concentrates on the medicinal and healing effects of the essential oil of the plant. In The Power of Flowers deck, my intention is to share the higher vibrational qualities of each flower, given to you in the form of a flower essence signature. It was this signature, or story, of the flower that inspired me to begin connecting human archetypes to the flowers. The living essence of the plant provoked in me the springing forth of visual beings who seemed to live within the flower's energy field. The flowers became more alive and accessible to me as I began to experience the quality of love held within the many archetypal images associated with them. I can imagine these beautiful beings assisting in the alchemical process of Flower Essence preparation and thus assisting in human evolution.

Art

Rudolph Steiner, a mystic and an educator in the early 1900's, spoke of the increasing need for art in culture. For, in his view, art and visual beauty stimulate "picture consciousness" within an individual. A skillful artist has the ability to unlock mysteries and imagination previously dormant within the human psyche, as well as to assist us in drawing upon the spiritual forces and angelic realms which overlight human intelligence and creativity. Whether the form of expression is painting, drawing, mosaic, stained glass, or some other medium, the opportunity always exists to see within a work of art the freedom and individuality of the artist.

During certain historical periods, artistic expression seems to achieve a rare brilliance, for it is in these times that individual genius and general evolutionary patterns accelerate to new heights. We are now living in such a time. This deck is a response to the collective need to visualize and heal through new means and modalities and to enliven our minds and hearts with artistic images that may move us to spiritual insight and new levels of development. Art that truly reflects the heart and soul of life can inspire us to dream new dreams and open anew to the possibility of the magical and the miraculous.

As already discussed, the preparation of flower essences is an alchemical art utilizing the golden rays of the sun, pure water, and flower blossoms. The elixir is complete when the pattern, or energy medicine, of the flower has been released into the water. With the aid of kirilian photography, beautiful shapes and designs are seen in each individual water droplet, revealing the unique qualities of the particular flower. Nature has various ways of showing Herself to us; often Her greatest mysteries are imprinted in our own souls in the form of refined energetic etchings, which we then seek to replicate. Ultimately, all art springs from nature, reflecting the shapes and colors found in the natural world. The seeker of spiritual truths is an artist; in profound ways, longing for the kind of artistic beauty and harmony that only Nature provides—cloaked, as She is, in the majesty of Flora, the consort of the flowers, and crowned with the stars of cosmic light. Humanity walks in the balance of nature's radiance, and the blossoming flowers of the Earth mirror the very essence of joy that is every person's birthright.

Color is a symphony heard throughout the rainbow spectrum. Flowers represent the blossoming of consciousness, for they are nature's rainbows. Likewise, the truest expression of the human soul is a rainbow body. For, ultimately, the soul is nothing other than a translucent, multi-colored field of pure consciousness, shimmering with feeling. The more conscious we become, the more brilliant and fluid are the colors of our auric rainbow. We need a full-color spectrum of possibilities in order to open the heart and stimulate joy and inspiration as we transmute through life's many challenges. In recognition of this fact, vibrant colors were chosen for The Power of Flowers cards. They depict the various colors of the soul as seen through the lens of the flower kingdom. They align us with a new awareness symbolized through archetypal imagery, accompanied by myths and stories. The cards serve as a doorway into the realm of imagination and personal attunement with nature. By focusing on their visual beauty and calling forth the healing that is revealed to you through images and colors, deep transformation is made possible.

Finally, in order to better convey the sublime teachings of the flower kingdom, Karen and I felt it was important to include human figures in the cards—representing the sacred aspects of certain archetypal themes. In this way, we can more readily relate to the higher vibratory patterns of the flowers, forming a strong, mystical link between humanity and nature. It is also known that faces and hands, as depicted in art, help connect humanity to the sacred. It is our hope that these images will reflect the divine grace of your innermost being, becoming an oracle of loving guidance for you.

Flower Application

Sunrise to sunset, flowers adorn our planet in a multitude of ways, and the subtle nature of their exquisite beauty is an eternal blessing to humanity. Even if you lived in a cave, and never actually saw a flower, they would still wrap you in their loving embrace, for the essence of flowers permeates the earth within and without. There are so many ways to engage with flowers, be it a stroll in the garden, a floral painting on the wall, scented oil from the blossoms, a bouquet of freshly picked flowers, or a vibrational remedy. We have the option of going to the flowers in any way we choose. My truest love, aside from the mere presence of the flowers themselves, is applying flower essence therapy. After twenty odd years of working with the elixirs, it is no longer about believing in them or proving that they work; I know them for the powerful healers they are. I know them as geometric poetry of the human soul. Each flower holds a specific healing pattern that is a miniature holographic universe of its own.

The primary purpose of the Power of Flower cards is to invite us to relate with nature more intimately through the practical application of flower essences. It is very important for people to understand that this is not a complicated science set aside for a gifted minority of mystically minded pioneers. The essences are here for all of humanity, rich or poor, and all color and creed. Edward Bach offered us a peek into the eternal medicine bag of nature, the plants themselves, asserting over and over again that the natural world speaks a language of harmony and goodwill for all of humankind. Bach wrote, "Once we realize our own Divinity, the rest is easy."

Flower essences address the conditions of both our spiritual and mortal bodies. If there is discord, disease will follow. Disease is the soul's way of addressing imbalance.

For example, negative emotions, such as fear and anger, create rigidity and disharmony in the body and these unhealthy constructs can eventually turn into physical disease. Flower essence therapy addresses the mental states within us that distort the soul's spiritual journey. Flower essences, working in the sacred space between body and soul, wash away our impurities, and anchor the soul in the rich new soil of encouragement and hope.

All people are invited to use flower essences in their everyday life in order to prevent and cure disease. We are all healers, graced with the virtues of love and compassion. It is the work of our souls to draw this force forward so as to be in service to one another. There are times, however, when a professional in the art of flower essence diagnosis can be of great service. One who has studied the flowers and observed the mental and emotional states of patients day in and day out may be able to diagnose flowers with great skill. One practitioner may use methods such as muscle testing and hypnotherapy to diagnose flowers, while another may use a pendulum. The most important tool of all, of course, is Love.

Through the laws of higher order, (regardless of our resistance), we are each graced with the potential to serve humanity. Likewise, we are offered the opportunity to align ourselves with a way of living that promotes respect for all individuals. The path to individuation is the key that unlocks the potential for each person to blossom and discover his or her path to freedom. Flower essences enable us to balance the mind so that we may overcome the human maladies and delusions that keep us from knowing the mission and destiny we have come to fulfill.

Flower essence application is varied and diverse, yet simple. Essences made from the living plants of our earth are imbued with a glorious luminosity, brimming with vitality and high vibrations. A vibrational medicine of the future, flower essence therapy may seem, at first glance, too simple to be true (especially to the western mind, trained as it is in the complexities of allopathic medicine). In fact, it was Edward Bach's wish, a wish he held until the day he died, to keep the art of flower essence therapy simple, pure, and available to all. He believed that the administering of essences should be as simple as walking out to the garden to pick some lettuce for your supper or hiking to the woods to pick mimulus for your fear. The bottled essences make it possible to reach for the guardians of nature through the apothecary of our own home. In this way, we may choose a flower helper to assist us in caring for ourselves and our loved ones.

I've been working with flower essences since 1976 and using the pendulum to diagnose flowers for the past fifteen years. While living at the Findhorn Foundation, I was introduced to the use of the pendulum by a man who used one to identify and diagnose energetic blockages related to the seven energy centers known as chakras. At first, I was leery of the pendulum because, in the area of spiritual exploration, I am quite cautious about new techniques until I feel a resonance within my own heart. Feeling drawn to the pendulum, I began experimenting with my own chakras and the energy field around my body. Next, I tried using the pendulum to determine which flower essences might be beneficial to me. It took a couple of years to get myself out of the way, to let the pendulum do its work, and to trust the process.

The most amazing thing about the diagnostic process is that empirical evidence will very often confirm that the flowers are on the right track. For example, someone might come in complaining of anxiety around a particular issue. This is the identified ailment. We'll discuss many aspects of the client's life and then we'll get out the pendulum and flower essences. Typically, the flowers will identify something much deeper living within the unconscious of the individual.

The pendulum responds to the electrical impulses of the body as it relates to the various flowers. Flower essences selected in this way can illuminate very subtle nuances concerning a person's overall health, including mental and emotional states. There are times when a client and I will be moved to tears as we surrender to the guidance of a Higher Will, and discover hidden aspects of the person's suffering that could not have been identified through our own rational processes alone.

Of course, it is possible to work very effectively with flower essences without the use of a pendulum. Each person must find his or her own way to relate skillfully with the healing essence of our floral allies.

All sentient beings benefit from the cures and elixirs nature has to offer. For example, flower application is used successfully with children, babies, animals, and plants.

The fact that it would be impossible to give a baby or an animal a bottle of essences, then suggest that they attune to the healing possibility it holds for them, demonstrates that essences are not a placebo (i.e. little bottles of high ideals and imagination).

It must be stated, however, that mental affirmations and thought constructs may very well have an effect on our healing. Additionally, an individual holding the image of health, radiance, and receptivity, may in fact, find better results with the flowers than one who holds rigid doubt and negativity. Flowers can be administered to deflect these conditions of pessimism and skepticism, as well.

There are many ways to apply the essences. The most common way is to take several drops orally, under the tongue, from a one ounce remedy bottle. This remedy is made by adding four to seven drops from the Mother Stock (this is the original essence made from the actual flowers and preserved in brandy) into a dropper bottle filled with spring water. Never use distilled or tap water. It is advised that you take the remedy at least four times a day.

It is especially lovely to take flower essences before sleep. For during dream time, they may stir the unconscious into new discovery, opening the soul to a panoramic world of inner visions.

Do not store your essence in hot or sunny places because they are highly sensitive. In addition, moldy particles can contaminate the remedy if it is not stored properly. It is best to store flower essences at room temperature or in a cool environment.

Applying essences topically is a way to energize particular areas of the body, including the seven major chakras. Massage therapists may add essences to the oils used for massage, or individual essences can be chosen for specific conditions and clients if the practitioner has brought the flowers into his or her practice.

Children benefit by having essences rubbed onto the bottom of their feet at night, especially if they do not want to take the essences orally. Essences may be added to juice, and, in this way also, given to babies and young children.

Place several drops of an essence into the palm of your hand to rub onto the fur of your pet. A little drop on your pet's nose is a fine way to administer to animals as they will lick the essences off immediately. Also, add the elixir to your animal's drinking bowl.

A bath made with essences and aroma therapy is an extra special way to treat yourself. It will sooth your soul in more ways than one. I highly recommend lavender essence with lavender bath oil for relaxation, or rose essence with rose bath oil and a bit of ylang ylang oil for a beautiful aphrodisiac. Adorn the sides of your bathtub with fresh rosemary or mint for an even greater sensation.

I use a spray bottle, the kind one would use to spray their indoor plants, to freshen my living space and office. A combination of crab apple (for cleansing) and pink yarrow (for sweet protection) keeps my space free from stagnant air. These are but a few suggestions from a long list of ways flower essences can be beneficial to your life.

Perhaps the greatest tragedy in life is to exist on this planet for an entire lifetime without ever having truly lived, and to die without the experience of having been truly born. It is important that we meet the many challenges of physical incarnation, that we surrender fully into the richness of experience which is part and parcel of earthly existence. When we finally surrender to that which we have been avoiding, we come to a place of peace and joy. Everlasting joy can be found when the path to our Self Realization, the journey to our core, includes the bitter and the sweet. Then we can join these two aspects of our life into a story of Wholeness.

Paradoxically, this surrender that I am advocating, is an act of will, of discipline, of intention. It is something that must be enacted over and over again, lest those deluded habits of mind reassert themselves. Just as a flower has a stem to hold itself erect, so we humans have our will force, the human stem. It is no accident that meditative traditions require us to keep our stem's straight and strong. How better to embrace whatever may arise in each new moment?

How better to unfold ourselves into this world? In the words of Rumi: How will you know the difficulties of being human, If you're always flying off to blue perfection? Where will you plant your grief-seeds? We need ground to scrape and hoe, Not the sky of unspecified desire.

The flowers and plants of the earth are sacred ground. Through the beauty of their healing may we become a mirror of their divinity, fully rooted in an earth body, yet forever reaching upward toward the conscious light of the sun, the aspect of our soul that illumines the path into the rainbow of our inner garden.

Chapter 2

Oracular Consciousness

And The Mythology of the Soul

Our birth is but a sleep and a forgetting:
the soul that rises with us, our life's star.

— Wordsworth

The ideal relationship between The Power of Flowers cards and one who seeks to use them wisely, is an alchemical dance in which the soul of the cards and the soul of the "reader" are synergistically attuned for the purpose of healing. For best results, a meditative frame of mind, prayerful attitude, and oracular consciousness must be brought to bear upon this sacred interaction. I cannot over-state the importance of combining these three elements—meditation, prayer, and oracular attunement— with the quest for new global awareness. We must use all of the tools at our disposal in order to align ourselves to the magnetic tone of the planet, which is, and will continue to be, to seek balance within nature and humanity.

As the title of this chapter suggests, its focus concerns the meaning and cultivation of "oracular consciousness" as it relates to the mythology of the soul. However, since med-itation and prayer are such an integral part of this alchemical equation, I offer a few words of explanation regarding their meaning and cultivation, as well. In the Bud-dhist frame of reference, one's Mind, or True Self, is like a deep, still ocean, on the surface of which impermanent waves of thought, feeling, and sensation continuously arise and perish, one after the other. This ocean of the Mind is inherently spacious, radiant, clear, awake, stable, pure, per-fect, limitless, and indestructible. Regular meditation, of the sort that helps one identify with these enlightened qualities, while emptying the Mind of all attachments and aversions is an indispensable basis for attuning to the oracular wisdom embodied in The Power of Flowers cards. Without this foundation, one's prayers and attunements will be subject to the myriad limitations of the ego. Once a meditative frame of reference has been established, such prayers and attunements can be held within its womb-like space, pregnant with all possibility.

The prayerful practice of asking for guidance and assistance from beings more spiritually evolved and powerful than ourselves, makes good common sense. Having the discernment and humility to recognize when we're in over our heads and need to ask for help is always a good thing. It's all about surrendering to our limitations as human/spiritual beings, knowing what resources are available to us, and using them wisely and with gratitude. In the interest of helping the reader tap into the healing resources of the Power of Flowers deck, I have included a blessing at the end of the explanation for each card.

Oracular attunement is similar to prayer in that it assumes a relationship to spiritually evolved beings from dimensions of reality other than our own. However, the nature of the relationship is somewhat different. Oracles are traditionally understood as wise ones who possess the gift of prophecy and divine storytelling—the mythology of the soul. We approach these sages for a very particular reason—so that together we might enter into the sacred realm of archetypal images and the stories or myths that derive from them. At the deepest possible level, we move beyond even these images, stories, and myths, however, to a direct experience of the primal energy which is their inspired source.

Mother Nature is the ultimate Oracle of The Power of Flowers cards, though she wears many faces, indicated by the thirty-two cards—each a variation on Her original theme. Through Her trees, flowers, herbs, stars, seeds, planets, and streams, She embodies Natura, the feminine soul of Nature. By our interactions with Nature's myriad forms, we are invited to comprehend the truth of our divinity, for hidden in Her creations are stored archetypal patterns of wisdom, healing, and oracular truth.

Human intelligence, and the ability to combine the faculties of feeling and thinking, are gifts we have been given as part of our birthright. Nature opens humanity to the feeling realm, beckoning us into the depths of contemplation and transformation. It is through intimate exposure to this realm, offering us levels of wisdom which go beyond the merely intellectual, that we return to the source, our True Selves, discovering therein the deepest attunement to our Universal Mother, or Anima Mundi. The Mother's guidance can only be put into divine service when the human heart and head—feeling and thinking—have come together, showing us the way to the temple of Higher truths. She guides us as we leap into the future where new myths, archetypes and truths are stored.

In ancient myth, the Virgin Isis sits in Her temple holding the secret teachings concerning the laws of nature. It is possible to visit Isis there, but one is not allowed to lift the veil which protects the mystery. However, the knowledge she carries is so much a part of who we truly, organically are, that if we fail to lift Her veil, we may not survive. If we find the courage to gaze into Her lovely face, we will be richly rewarded, for we will have caught a glimpse of our own True Face, as well.

When we study the mythology of the great Goddesses and Gods, we discover that such myths are always embedded in natural cycles of birth, death, and rebirth—for like nature, archetypes embody the birth and death cycles we must learn to embrace if we are to continue to evolve. The human archetypes I have chosen for this project are mythical figures who function as powerful mirrors of the human soul. Each in their own way, they strengthen our courage to lift the veils, so that we may behold the potential of our own soul. When one is able to remove the veil, one is greeted by the great Oracle, and set free to explore the hidden mysteries of nature, as well as of one's self. For the separation of nature and humanity no longer exists. Once this false separation is overcome, the truth about nature's patterns, cycles, gestures, colors, scents, and sounds is readily perceived and understood. To achieve Oracular Consciousness—attunement to the mystery which is no longer a mystery—is to be divinely inspired and guided by the Goddess Natura.

We must awaken to a path here on Earth where the folds of Natura's garment can again be touched. The time is now. If we truly want to know Her—we must gather the courage and humility to look into the dark places within ourselves and bring them to the light. This is the oracular work of alchemy, where opposites combine in order to bring about transformation. The more we learn, the more humble we become. New information is revealed, and new streams of consciousness flow into our hearts.

Knowledge must remain fluid, for once it hardens and solidifies, it no longer lives within the soul. The many images that reside in our soul and higher mind are carried along by a stream of consciousness which has never stopped flowing, for even a moment, throughout eternity. Mythologies of ancient and future times are the stories and images of our soul, transferred to us from a place of cosmic truth and love. As we open to the Oracle within, we discover pictures and stories that stimulate our willingness to do our inner work. The information we receive may present us with many challenges, but it will also prove an invaluable resource in the quest for self-realization.

It is imperative that we bring myth and Oracular mindfulness together in order to prepare our minds for truth in whatever form it presents itself: as a great Goddess; a beautiful flower; or a work of art. Picture stories and myths are a form of healing and Oracular teaching stemming from the earliest imprints of our souls' collective yearning. Symbols, signs, patterns, designs of nature—all are revealed through art. In combining the mysteries of nature with the mythology of the human soul, we generate new symbols and imagery, guiding us down the path of inspiration, imagination and continued development.

Not far from dreams, myths point to the metaphoric consciousness of humanity, showing the living structure of the psyche. Through immersion in the mythological realm, we encounter the holy aspects of this inner domain. Here is where myth is born. The mythology of the soul represents our historic quest for understanding, which is at the core of the evolution of consciousness. Heroes, heroines, saints, Gods, Goddesses—all arise out of the need for deeper knowledge, as well as a context within which to work through the many challenges of being human.

Mythic figures listen and respond to the call from other dimensions. They show us the way to our spiritual life, which is a constant adventure—a vision quest. Nature, the moon, the sun, the plants and trees, play an integral part in helping us create, discover, and reinvent our myths—the pictures by which we identify the core meaning of life—for nature has many stories to tell. Plants and trees carry a myriad of clues in the very structure of their beings which can be read or interpreted by anyone who is willing to listen.

Studying the unique form of each flower, actualizes the mythology of the plant and reveals the God or Goddess residing within. Each flowers is a jewel arising from the depth of the seed—its secret revealed in the blossoming potential of growth and development. As the plant progresses through cycles of death and rebirth, its flower and fruit give their seeds of wisdom back to the earth in order to once again germinate toward a new beginning.

With The Power of Flowers cards, the artist, Karen Forkish, and I, the creatress and author, wish to explore the flowering potential of archetypes and mythical beings as they mirror and reflect the miracle of our temporal existence. The cards in this project were created with the hope that they may each become a mini temple which you may enter in order to receive Nature's esoteric teachings. Whether you meet QuanYin, the fairy spirits, or Krishna, may you continue to ensoul through their model of higher inspiration and perfection.

Chapter 3

How To Use The Cards

Divine Play and Enchantment

When you find a poem or a picture that really
appeals to you, and awakens you, there is
someone who went ahead of you and gives you
that experience; and it may be life-shaping.

— Joseph Campbell

The Power of Flowers cards are a dynamic convergence of art, nature, myth, and healing, a fervent prayer with the ability to inspire surrender to the mystery of nature as a "living garden"—a New World Paradise. They were created primarily out of a deeply felt desire to assist in the restoration of nature's divine graces so that such graces might enchant humanity and illuminate the path toward Self-love and enlightenment.

In fairy tales and folklore, the term "enchantment" relates to the mystery that must be solved within a story, be it through a dream, a deep sleep, a wish, a task, a trance, or even an hallucination. Enchantment has accomplished its alchemical work when the heroine or hero is transformed and awakened into a new vision or way of being, thus carrying the treasures of new consciousness into a new life. This is the "flowering potential" of the fable, for hidden qualities of joy are released, freeing one from slumber and suffering. Ultimately, enchantment is indicative of a major transition, where rebirth is accomplished out of the incubating seeds of love, hope, and clarity.

The cards that you hold in your hands were created to assist you in reinventing the stories that live within your body and soul. This is so that you might move beyond the limits of mortal confinement, and leap into the magical world of "enchantment." The Iris can whisk you into a land of lush, rainbow transformation, showing you the way to creative fulfillment. The Poppy beckons you to dreamtime, where you meet the guardians of your soul; while the Pomegranate ushers in the underworld, where treasures of self-knowledge are stored, making their retrieval possible. Finally, the Violet embodies the divinity of women, leading both men and women upward on a new path to the regeneration of the Pure Feminine within.

Toward the ultimate goal of enchantment, The Power of Flowers cards have many practical uses and applications. For example, an image chosen at any given moment may inspire a vision quest of sorts and bring to life the living qualities of the flower, its essence, and its archetypal companion. Placing the card on an altar or sacred space in the home can magnify the essential meaning of the card in your everyday life, for the image will begin to "flower" within the soul as a fertile potential. Likewise, the flower represented in a card can be put in a vase near the chosen image, invoking the presence of nature and assisting one's communication with the higher intelligence of the plant. Also, the use of flower remedies and elixirs is highly recommended. They are sold in most health food stores or can be ordered (see Flower Essence Resource Directory in back). Placing drops of the flower tincture under the tongue is a powerful way to be healed and energized by the plant's medicine.

Another effective method for using the cards is to meditate on the visual image depicted, allowing the image to permeate your heart and third eye. When we study the form or visual image of a flower, we are, in fact, reading its very soul, for the myth of the plant is organically embedded in nature. For example, Lady Slippers tell us by their shape that they are a remedy for foot disorders, while Cat's Ears hint at their effectiveness in treating hearing loss. Sunflowers, which spiral boldly toward the Sun only to bow in humility upon reaching their destination, assist in the alchemical marriage of masculine and feminine principles. And, roses, with their incredibly deep roots, teach us about the staying power of unconditional love, the deepest love of all.

Visualization techniques, such as mandala art and color therapy are potent tools that help to align and balance chakras, meridian points, and the auric field. Each flower vibrates to a specific color and energy charge, serving as a healing current that electrifies the human body. For instance, red flowers will have a vitalizing effect upon the individual, where a purple flower will attune one to spiritual aspirations. You may wish to concentrate on the feeling of the card in order to discover how it stimulates or comforts the psyche. When we listen with our hearts, the flowers, art, and symbolism will carry us into the music and harmony of our spirit. The cards can also invoke one's connection to holy places and sacred prayer.

Hold the cards during meditation in order to transfer higher vibrations to them, energizing the relationship between the flowers, the archetypes, and yourself. Choosing an image while in a deeply meditative state of grace allows one to commune with the healing of the card in profound ways. In times of crisis, spiritual emergence or emergency (sometimes the line between these two is very thin), or illness, the cards can be utilized as a healing Oracle. Flower essences are especially beneficial when our bodies are out of balance on the emotional, physical, spiritual, and mental planes. The archetypal image associated with the flower may have a crucial message concerning the improving of one's health.

Celebrations, called "rites of passage," are enjoying a resurgence of popularity in our culture, adorned with fresh ideas interwoven with the old. A young girl or boy reaching the age of puberty is sometimes honored by elders, mothers, fathers, siblings, and friends. The Power of Flowers cards can enhance such an event by lending the beauty and grace of Nature and Her message to the ceremony. These precious transitions honor the "blossoming beauty" of the individual, strengthening self-confidence, courage, and integrity, as our young people meet the world with love and support.

Spread the cards in a large circle, face down, and place a candle and a bouquet of roses and orchids in a beautiful vase at the center. The candle flame signifies purification, illumination, and light; the flowers symbolize the guardians of the soul. More specifically, the roses represent unconditional love and deep divinity, emphasizing the Divine Feminine, while the orchids represent spiritual will and sexuality, harmonizing and balancing the Divine Masculine. The merging of these two flowers symbolize the inner marriage of the feminine and masculine, activating the alchemical marriage within the soul of the individual, and stimulating awareness and wholeness as one ventures into the world of relationships.

The young initiate will be asked to choose a card from the circle. The flower image chosen serves as a representative of the overlighting protection that surrounds and encourages the progress of the soul's journey. The young person should be encouraged to share his or her impressions and feelings about the card before the book is opened and read. Each member of the group or circle will then choose a card, offering the grace of its symbol and message. After each participant has shared their card, the deck is put back into a single pile and offered to the child as a special gift—a cherished memory of a crucial time of transition. Similar ceremonies can be held for many transitional celebrations, such as: the birth of a new baby; an elder's rite of passage into crone/sage status, birthdays, New Year's day, or passages into death and dying.

Layout patterns are a more extensive and involved way to receive guidance and inspiration through the cards. You are, of course, encouraged to invent your own layouts. In addition, the following unique Power of Flowers card readings have been created for use during times of self-reflection, healing, and celebration.

The Soul's Garden

Within each individual, there is a sacred place to which one must periodically retreat for guidance and insight. This inner journey delivers us into the deep recesses of the psyche, where magic and wisdom can be found. This layout is a one card message. Fan the cards upright so that all of the flowers are visible, representing the beautiful garden within. Allow the intuitive (non-dominant) hand to scan the landscape of colorful images before you until one of the flowers is picked—just as you have at some time in your life been inspired to pick a real flower from an earthly garden.

A flower picked from a garden needs water in order to sustain its life force. In turn, the card which you have picked has qualities which can nurture you, and, in a sense, water the roots of your own core self. Use your well-tuned instincts as you align to the gifts offered through your chosen flower.

32 Cards Fanned

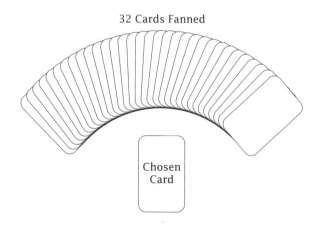

Chosen
Card

Flowers of Love

The Power of Flower Cards wish to speak to the grace and beauty of the flowering creative spirit living in the cave of your heart. This Flower Self (High Self) holds the memory of your origins and speaks through the lens of Eternal Love, uniting with the wisdom of the Earth which lives within you—just as the tender part of your spirit stands on sacred ground, feeling the earth as a living being. Recalling and honoring this aspect of the Self can help realign you with plants, healing work, creativity, and joyous service. This, in turn, can lead to ecstatic feelings about the entire world.

First, the cards are spread into a circle representing the womb from which all love springs forth. From the circle, choose four cards representing the letters L O V E and place them face down in the center. Turn the cards up one at a time starting with the letter "L." The first card, "L," represents the Life qualities and gifts that you are given at birth. Next, "O" represents the Open Channel through which you are able to speak your truth. The "V" represents the Victory which will result as you identify and begin to fulfill your divine purpose. Finally, "E" represents Eternity, your Everlasting blessing and prayer.

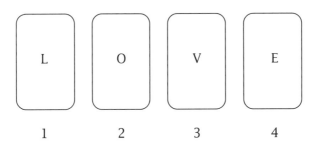

The Blossoming Self

Every day we are surrounded by the miracles of nature, be it a spring that never tires of providing fresh water, the Sun that warms us each day, or the multitudes of fragrant flowers that grace our Earth. Nature provides an endless and abundant source of protection, inspiration, and nurturance. This reverent power tugs at the soul of humanity, reminding us that we are living temples, walking amongst nature like human flowers, pouring forth our love and wisdom to all we encounter. They offer this gentle yet persistent reminder so that we may understand that we are not separate from the awesome beauty that embraces us.

This layout is a mirror, a divine picture of your flowering Self, in full bloom and radiant. The five cards are positioned in the shape of a flower. The number five representing the creative qualities of spiritual development which reflect the infinite and benevolent nature of

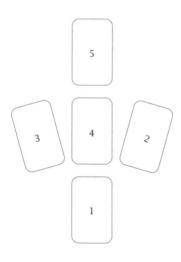

your True Self. Card #1 represents the root and core of one's inner reality, all that sustains one's life, including the ancestral patterns from which we emerge. Card #2 represents the sprouting leaf of consciousness that is prominent and fully recognized in a person's life, offering a glimpse of personal illumination and clarification. Card #3 represents the leaf of unconscious growth that is yet to be discovered within the sanctuary of the individual and mirrors the qualities that are ready to blossom and emerge. Card #4 represents the stem that carries these potentials to the glorification of personal achievement and success. Card #5 represents the crowning attainment of Self. The image presented to the individual serves as a source of inspiration and hope, for these are the aspiring talents and gifts that are soon to be recognized and experienced in one's daily life.

Flowers are songs as much as they are prayers. Dancing spirits of nature, they invite us to partake of their joy, greeting us as angelic messengers who hold the patterns of heavenly secrets and teachings within their fragrant, earthly blossoms. The flowers and archetypes represented in this reading seek to embrace you with a pure heart.

Flower Chakra Healing

In nature, the spiral is sacred. Its pattern of movement portrays the mystical notion that what begins shall end and thus begin again. The spiral is found in nature as follows: the first tender shoots and sprouts that break free from the seed; root formations deep in the earth; sea shells with their intricate circular patterns; flower blossoms; spiraling water in a river's current; and the spinning chakras of the human energy centers. Labyrinthian designs were also common in cathedrals, temples, and sacred sites, representing the natural cycles of death and rebirth which were symbolically walked by initiates as they moved through the gates of "eternity."

In the human body, there are seven spiraling energy centers, known as chakras. They carry spiraling energy, or kundalini, from the base of the spine toward the pinnacle, the crown chakra (located at the top of the head), radiating this energy outward until it descends again into the rebirth of a new cycle. They supply the creative fire or life force our bodies need for self-healing and regeneration. Concentrating on the maintenance and health of the seven chakras can maximize one's capacity to stay in excellent condition on all levels.

This layout offers information concerning your health, security, creativity, and spiritual alignment. The diagram indicates where each of the chakras are located in the body and identifies key points corresponding to each energy center. After shuffling and attuning to the cards, lay the chosen seven cards in a vertical line beginning with the # 1 card, representing the 1st chakra, at the bottom. Each card will reveal the issues related to each particular chakra. You may wish to rub the flower essences associated with each card externally on the chakra center to which it is connected, while meditating on the message that comes to you, allowing the healing to penetrate deep into the cells of your body.

First Chakra: This energy center is located at the base of the spine and governs all issues related to safety, security, and the survival life force. It is represented by the color red. Key question: How do I empower my life force.

Second Chakra: This energy center is located two fingers below the navel and governs the creative and procreative powers. Issues related to sexuality, self-expression, and deep tissue memory are stored here. It is represented by the color orange. Key question: How do I empower my creativity and self- expression?

Third Chakra: This energy center is located at the center of the body between the navel and the rib cage and is most identified as the solar plexus.

Issues related to personal integrity, honor, and self-confidence are connected to this point. It is represented by the color yellow. Key question: Do I live according to my higher integrity and individuation?

Fourth Chakra: This is the heart chakra. Issues related to love, emotion, and feelings are connected to this primary center of human energy. It is represented by the color green. Key question: Do I love others and myself unconditionally?

Fifth Chakra: This is the throat chakra. Issues related to speech, safety in self-expression and clarity are activated. It is represented by the color blue. Key question: Do I speak in truth and clarity about my life and my needs?

Sixth Chakra: This is the center known as the Third Eye located at the center of the forehead. Issues related to intuition, dreams, visions, and higher understanding are associated with this point. It is represented by the color purple. Key question: Am I receptive to the guidance of my High Self?

Seventh Chakra: This is the center known as the Crown chakra located at the top of the head and extends several inches above the head. This is the connecting point with the first chakra and is the point that balances heaven with Earth, or, As Above, So Below. It is the contact point to our Angelic Self and enhances meditation, visualization, prayer, and Higher Knowledge. The color white or indigo represents it. Key question: Do I honor and integrate my God/Goddess Self in my every day life?

Layouts are there to create a map or outline from which you may create an intention to bring new meaning and understanding to your life. They offer a guideline from which to survey the Inner Self. It is equally powerful to use the cards in any way you wish, just as long as they are cared for and respected. Here is a list of options:

Choose one card to reflect a situation, person, or decision.

Use these cards to enhance other readings with other decks. For example, you may wish to over light a tarot reading with a Power of Flower card in order to discover the archetypal energy that is with you and the message.

Use the cards during a flower essence consultation and learn what the message the flowers hold for you.

Use them during rituals and blessings. Have each person choose a card as a blessing.

Enjoy them, and let them into your heart.

Flower Chakra Healing

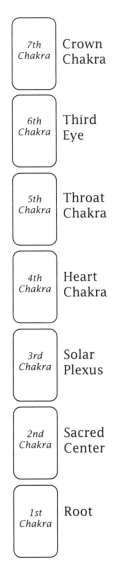

7th Chakra — Crown Chakra

6th Chakra — Third Eye

5th Chakra — Throat Chakra

4th Chakra — Heart Chakra

3rd Chakra — Solar Plexus

2nd Chakra — Sacred Center

1st Chakra — Root

The Power of Flowers

Card Descriptions

Rose

LATIN: Rosaceae

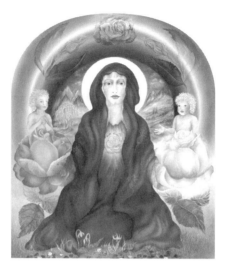

Blessing

Holy Rose, Queen of Love,
Your beauty is Divine.
Sacred is your tenderness,
Jewel of nature,
Sweet and kind.

Plant Signature

The rose family includes many species of five-petaled flowers in the shape of pentagrams, or five-pointed stars, which offer humanity a beautiful symbol of Cosmic Love accessible through the human heart. The rose's thorny stem is in marked contrast to its sweet scent, reflecting the suffering and pain one must sometimes endure in order to understand and experience real love. Perhaps humanity will one day evolve beyond the need for thorns, but for now "more suffering is evidently necessary."

The roots of the rose bush grow deep into the ground, making the uprooting of this plant difficult. Just as a human being can surmount great obstacles, especially with the purity of Self-Love as a foundation, the rose bush is tenacious and can endure extreme weather and neglect.

Flower Essence

The rose essence is one of the purest vibrations in existence. Whatever its color or species, it always invokes the most profound dimensions of love—accomplishing this through a gentle stimulation of the heart chakra, located at the center of the human body. Perhaps the rarest and most sublime of all rose essences is derived from the green rose. It opens the heart chakra, which is strengthened by the color green, to extremely high levels of intuition channeled through the very core of the human heart.

Archetype
MADONNA; MARY, QUEEN OF HEAVEN, MOTHER OF THE WORLD

The Virgin Mary has, at various times, been referred to as The Holy Rose, the Mystic Rose, and Goddess of the Rose. The rosary, or "rose wreath," originating in the Middle East as a form of worship to the Virgin Goddess, was eventually Christianized, taking the form of a prayer to the Virgin Mary. What is more, it has been said that Mary's immaculate conception was brought about by a magic rose. Similarly, it was not uncommon for stained glass windows in ancient Christian cathedrals to depict Mary surrounded by roses.

Like the five-petaled apple blossom and the five-lobed apple, the rose forms a natural pentagram. While the apple is associated with Aphrodite, Goddess of Love, as well as with Eve in the Garden of Eden, its close counterpart, the rose, is associated with Mary, said to be The Second Eve and also known as The Flower of Venus.

It was in ancient India that the Goddess was first symbolized as The Holy Rose whose body was considered a temple. This philosophy gave rise to an understanding that the temple, the garden, and the female body were mystically one, coalescing into the pure, fertile womb of regeneration. In later Gnostic cathedrals, the Goddess was represented as the Universe itself, containing the essence of the male, or the masculine principle, within herself.

At the mystical core of Christianity, Mary, a derivative of the Goddess, embodies the immaculate mystery of birth, for her Christ child represents the alchemical balance of masculine and feminine principles which issue forth from her womb. Mary, the Moon, gives birth to The Light of the World in the form of the Cosmic Child, making her the Cosmic birther of all that is sacred. Sadly, our culture has lost its connection to this deeper mythology of the "Queen of Heaven."

Healing

The Austrian mystic Rudolph Steiner offers a unique perspective on the birth of Christ, suggesting that Mary, in fact, gave birth to twin souls: one dedicated to the path of the Truth, the yellow rose; and the other dedicated to the path of the Heart, the pink rose. In this way, according to Steiner, Mary offered the world both the forces of Universal Logos and of Universal Love.

In choosing this card, you are greeted by the Rose Goddess, gently announcing your readiness to accept the twin gifts of Cosmic Love and Wisdom embodied by the Mystic Rose. Mary's balancing of the head and the heart is symbolized by the Sun, aglow as an aura of Light around her head, and an illumined rose, shining forth from deep within her heart. Behind her stands a weeping willow tree offering its branches to mystical muses for the making of wands. Such branches were once considered cosmic connectors to the stars. Mary sits surrounded by the delicate flower Shooting Star. The flower essence derived from its blossoms assists humanity with the birthing of higher forms of consciousness on Earth.

Allow your mind to be illumined with the yellow clarity of the Sun as you open your Solar Body to new inspiration. At the same time, open your heart to the stream of rose light now encircling your energy field. You are dearly blessed.

Practical Application

The Rose is considered the lotus of the heart. Its vibration is pure and devotional, offering a full spectrum of colors, each a variation on the general theme. For example: the White Rose purifies the heart; the Pink Rose gently opens and protects the heart; the Yellow Rose bridges mind and heart; the Red Rose strengthens the vein of love between two people and deepens the romantic quality of the heart; the Peach Rose offers peace and gaiety to the heart; and, finally, multi-colored roses blend and mix the variations described above.

The Rose essence is one of the most beneficial for conditions of the heart, the heart chakra, and issues regarding love. Highly effective when taken by itself, the healing properties of this essence can be greatly enhanced when used in tandem with Rose oil or aroma therapy. You may blend the Rose flower elixir with massage oil or lotion and gently rub it around the heart chakra. Several of my clients report visions of incandescent pink or white light surrounding them when they are massaged with Rose essence.

The Rose essence unites with the Universal Feminine Matrix, and, consequently, I have connected it to the Divine Mother. Therefore, I suggest that my clients hang or carry with them a picture or a symbol of the Divine Mother from the tradition of their choice, and that as they take the essence, they visualize their lives graced with the over lighting presence of Her Unconditional Love. Likewise, when aligning yourself to the Rose and its healing properties, I suggest you anchor and attune yourself to Mother Earth, for She holds the roots of this beloved plant deep within Her, just as the Rose essence grounds and sustains your healing.

When my youngest daughter, Sophie, was born, a dear friend planted a Wild Rose in our yard in celebration of her birth. This plant has blossomed with tremendous abundance year after year, showering my daughter with indescribable love and protection. Each spring since she has been old enough to understand, Sophie goes out into the yard eager to see if there are new buds on the plant, and at six years old, she now comes running to tell me how much love the flowers are giving her. When she is sad, she is often drawn to the rose bush for consolation, as well. I highly recommend planting a rose bush for a new baby. It is a beautiful way to honor a child, offering tangible yet magical Love from the realm of the flowers.

Rose is also a beautiful essence for use during pregnancy and childbirth. It can be rubbed onto the belly, enhancing the quality of Love exchanged between mother and unborn child. I recommend putting a drop of Rose essence, highly diluted, on the rosy lips of the newborn, welcoming him or her with perhaps the sweetest elixir on Earth.

Pomegranate

LATIN: Punica granatum

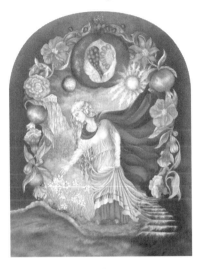

Blessing

Pomegranate ushers us down to meet,
The Sacred Feminine and Her seeds so sweet,
Bearing fruit, luscious and red,
Into Her Labyrinth,
I am led.

Plant Signature

The flower of the Pomegranate buds in oval, womb-shaped orbs. When fully opened, a deep red flower with a yellowish center and a core of tiny seeds is revealed. The fruit is quite unique with hard dry skin and a nest of bright red juicy seeds within—making it a natural symbol for female fertility.

Flower Essence

We sometimes lose touch with core feelings and misguid-edly seek to meet our inner needs outside the scope of balanced soul integration. Pomegranate essence restores self-nurturing qualities to the individual by assisting in the identification of deep, long-buried, emotional needs, especially in relation to the mother, childbearing, and creative issues. Gently, this essence guides us to the womb of the second chakra, the energy center located two inches below the navel where procreative forces are focused in the human body. In this way, it restores and regenerates fertility on all levels, beautifully attuning us to Mother Love in the process.

Archetype

PERSEPHONE, KORE, QUEEN OF THE UNDERWORLD

The fable of Kore, Queen of the Underworld, predates the Greek version in which Kore, now known as Persephone, is abducted by Pluto and held hostage in the Underworld. In the original version, Kore is worshipped as Goddess of the Blessed Dead, for it is believed that she holds the keys to the lower worlds as well as to the heavens, and can journey to the jeweled center of the Earth to cultivate the fertile seeds stored within its core.

As Persephone, she is the daughter of Demeter, the Great Mother, who resides at the center of the Triple God-dess Trinity comprised of Maiden, Mother, and Crone. With the abduction of Persephone to the Underworld, Demeter is grief-stricken. In her grief, she banishes all fruit, flower, and grain from the face of the Earth. This action is symbolic, for Demeter represents the rage we sometimes feel when dra-matic changes—such as menopause, childbirth, the death of a loved one, or the temporary loss of our identity—occur in our lives. Deep cycles and rhythms of birth and death per-meate the inner world of our psyches, surfacing at such powerful moments of initiation.

Persephone signifies the renewed aspect of self that is to be found if only we are willing to travel into the chambers of rebirth in order to gather the seeds of new possibilities. While in the nether regions, she gathers the six-petaled Narcissus, flower of the Underworld. Then, as Persephone prepares to resurface, returning to the light of her Mother's garden, representing the conscious world, she consumes six Pomegranate seeds which enable her to remain above ground for six months of the year. Her joyful reunion with Demeter heralds not only Spring, but ultimately the triumph of Life over Death.

Persephone's cyclic journey between the forces of birth and death mirrors that of the Black Madonna in the Celtic mysteries. Until the French Revolution when it was destroyed, a statue in the Madonna was kept deep in the chambers of Chartres Cathedral for the six darkest months of the year. Each Spring when the days became longer, she would be taken out of the darkness in a symbolic celebration of rebirth and renewal. In rituals of this sort, all that is heavy or weighed down in the soul is allowed to blossom upward toward the Sun's radiance.

Healing

On her journey, Persephone is protected by the luminaries, the Sun and the Moon. She knows that the gestating seeds within her will open to the sunlight even as they are watered by the changing cycles of the Moon.

Persephone is your guide. Standing between fire and water, she gazes into the beauty of Narcissus. As a bridge between the worlds, you, like Persephone, are forever crowned Queen of the Underworld, and, yet, eternally nourished by the love and mystery of Mother Earth. She will protect you as you make your descent in order to discover for yourself the splendor and magic of the mysterious forces within.

Practical Application

Pomegranate essence has been one of the most successful elixirs in my practice with women. Flower essences are vibrational essences, and are not often used to heal actual physical disorders, although they do assist in breaking through the patterns that eventually create disease in the body. However, Pomegranate as a vibrational essence seems to produce immediate affect on the physical body. Associated with Persephone and the inner labyrinth, this essence mirrors the inner cavern of a woman's body, the womb—the sanctuary for the ultimate creative process. If there are blockages in this area of the body, many disorders can result, including ovarian cysts, menstrual irregularities, PMS, infertility, and other female maladies. Pomegranate heals these blocked areas, allowing the seeds of procreativity to revitalize.

I offer this remedy to clients who are seeking to consciously conceive a child, as it aids in fertility and receptivity. For example, when a client by the name of Suzanne was distraught over her inability to conceive after multiple attempts, I recommended Pomegranate, Fig, and Rose essence for her, suggesting that she bathe in the Pomegranate essence while visualizing the ripe, luscious fruit nurturing her body. Three weeks later, an ecstatic Suzanne phoned to give me the good news. She was pregnant! This is but one of many, many instances in which Pomegranate has helped heal a woman's reproductive system. When used in conjunction with Mugwart flower essence, I have seen Pomegranate regulate a woman's menstrual cycle on a number of occasions. Without question, it has helped to restore health and vitality in many women's lives, including my own.

This remedy is useful for men, as well, for it helps to retrieve and develop the ability to nurture. Not surprisingly, it also seems to help heal a man's relationship with his mother, especially if the relationship was damaged by a lack of maternal nurturance. Pomegranate moistens the Soul with the sweet milk of Mother Love, soothing the grief caused by hardened emotions.

Lotus

LATIN: *Nelumbo nucifera*

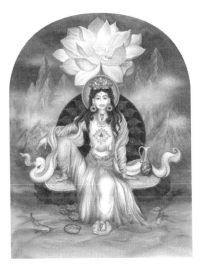

Blessing

Divine Lotus,
Your thousand petaled blossom ignites,
Spiritual rebirth and keen insight,
In silent bliss,
In infinite Love,
I embody your Wisdom,
From above.

Plant Signature

The lotus is a water plant with roots reaching deep into the muddy earth. Its pastel pink, yellow-centered petals close each night as the moon appears in the night sky, only to arise each morning as the Sun ushers in a new day. In the center of the flower is a capsule containing thousands of nut-like seeds capable of sprouting after laying dormant for centuries. According to Hindu cosmology, before Creation, the world was a Golden Lotus known as Matripadma, the Mother Lotus, or Womb of Nature.

Flower Essence

As an elixir, the Lotus stimulates Divine Inspiration and Spiritual Liberation. Miraculously, it moves the dark and muddy aspects of the psyche upward, ultimately enabling them to self-liberate through the crown chakra, the seventh sacred center of the body. The Lotus assists us in receiving guidance and insight from spiritual realms and can strengthen meditative states of consciousness wherein wisdom and tranquillity are to be found. This sacred flower should be used with much humility and gratitude, for it is a great help to humanity at this time of spiritual crisis.

Archetype
QUAN-YIN

Quan-yin, known as the Mother of Compassion, is the Buddhist embodiment of compassionate, skillful means. Having formerly been a male deity by the name of Avalokitesvara, she underwent a sex change in ancient China because it was thought that only the feminine principle could adequately inspire and guide spiritual seekers to the terrifying abyss known as emptiness—the great unknown where the ego drops away and there is only "one's original face before you were born," the True Self. For her great skill in this regard, she is likened to the Lotus.

To the Gnostic Christians, she was known as the Holy Spirit or World Mother, and was said to have ushered in the Golden Balance residing in the hearts of all people.

Healing

In the East, the Lotus is considered a perfect microcosmic reflection of the growth of human consciousness through three stages of evolution: ignorance; skillful means, and enlightenment. At the first stage, corresponding to ignorance, the Lotus roots extend upward from the muddy lake bottom. At the second stage, corresponding to skillful means, the Lotus stem is caressed and supported by the water. Finally, at the third stage, corresponding to enlightenment, the Lotus flower blossoms into the light of day.

Quan-Yin comes to you at this moment to reassure and inspire you in your spiritual quest for full awakening. As a bodhisattva of infinite compassion, She appears to you in whatever form will most aid you on your journey. Your yearning for enlightenment is witnessed, honored and fulfilled.

Quan-Yin sits on the Thousand Petaled Throne, the tantric symbol for the "yoni," or feminine principle. She honors the waters of life, the Great Womb of Suchness, wherein all beings reside—whether in ignorance or in an enlightened state. Pregnant with all possibilities, She makes even the most profound realization possible, and no one awakens without embracing Her feminine nature in the process. This card signifies spiritual birth. The vessel at Quan-yin's side is a gift of Her mysteries offered to you. You are crowned with the Thousand Petaled Lotus for many seeds of wisdom are germinating within you. What new level of realization are you about to birth?

Practical Application

The Lotus Elixir must be used with great reverence, for it attunes one to the seventh chakra, or crown, and opens the channels of the chakras above the head vertically aligned with your High Self.

Thus, it facilitates the grounding of higher knowledge, meditative experience and spiritual vision. When seeking this type of assistance, you might rub some of this essence directly onto the crown chakra (do not do this if you plan to drive or operate heavy machinery, however!). You might also drop some of the elixir in a warm bath, listen to beautiful music, and attune your Self to Quan-Yin. You will become like a thousand petaled lotus in the water, flowering and opening to higher states of awareness as the muddy depths of your unconscious are cleansed, refreshed and purified.

Clients engaged in the study of spiritual traditions and disciplines often benefit from the use of the Lotus elixir. For example, Sara, a graduate student in Religious Studies, used the Lotus essence while writing her dissertation on Buddhist themes related to the 12-Step Recovery model. Consequently, she reported an ability to think in more subtle and nuanced terms about the interplay of these two spiritual paths.

Lotus essence also attunes one to new cycles of spiritual attainment and has helped many clients access greater clarity regarding their true life missions. A client named Cynthia came to me feeling confused and lost in the midst of a mid-life crisis centered around her career. Later, she described being gently led to a place of clarity and surrender to her destiny while under the healing influence of this powerful elixir. In retrospect, she described really knowing all along what she was here to accomplish but pretending not to know due to feelings of unworthiness. With the help of the Lotus essence, the veil of unworthiness was parted long enough for Cynthia to remember her true self, and to find new direction and the motivation and energy to move forward. Much to her delight, Cynthia discovered that everything she had previously learned or experienced, even those events that had seemed accidental or random, was, in fact, part of some bigger plan preparing her for her life's work. Absolutely nothing was wasted.

When creating a sacred healing circle for ritual purposes, Lotus essence may be added to a bowl of water placed at the center of the circle. Put a white candle beside the bowl and ask that the flame of purification burn as all members of the circle bless themselves with the water, dabbing it on their foreheads, hearts, and the palms of their hands. Next, each person may move the energy of purification around the body, encircling the aura, cleansing it and freeing it of mental, emotional, physical, and spiritual blockages. The entire room will soon be filled with light as each person bathes in the nectar of the Lotus essence. A statue of Quan-Yin may be present, for She is the consort who guides one through the gates of purification. In fact, I often wash my statue of Quan-Yin in a Lotus bath. She emanates such love and beauty after the cleansing, I recommend the same to others.

Iris

LATIN: Iridaceae

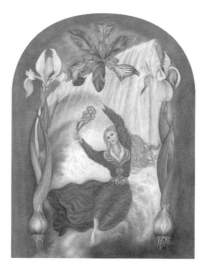

Blessing
Queen of Rainbow, Iris bright,
Pour forth your creative rays of light,
As we dance, As we sing,
We rejoice in the waters,
Of your Eternal Spring.

Plant Signature

The Iris family contains over sixty genera and perhaps 1000 species. Often found growing wild on the edge of a pond or stream, the Iris is a perennial herb with long, narrow, sword-shaped leaves, and rhizomes, or bulb-like rootstocks. With three petals, three sepals, and three stamen, its growth pattern is symbolically related to the power of the trinity, in particular, as well as to ever-changing cycles, in general. The beardless Iris represented here flourishes if constantly covered with water in early Spring.

Flower Essence

The Iris essence is extraordinarily beautiful and serves as a rainbow bridge between earth and sky, body and soul, and the temporal and spiritual worlds, reminding us of our infinite creativity and divine origins. Offering the expression of its ever-flowing form, it nourishes the human soul, unblocks old patterns of self-limitation and stagnation, inspires one to the heights of beauty and grace, and restores a path to art and creativity. The uncultivated Iris, found on the moist, forest floor, is the most potent variety of Iris to use for an essence. The garden variety makes for a wonderful essence, too, however, and can be collected from the early morning dew drops forming a pool at the center of its flower.

Archetype
IRIS—THE RAINBOW GODDESS

In Greek mythology, Iris, Queen of the Gods, was the Goddess of the Rainbow and Messenger of Hera. She traveled freely between the lower realms and the realm of the Gods, sometimes borrowing mortal shape, sometimes manifesting in her divine beauty and form—always offering an elixir of mercy and kindness, beauty and love, to those she met. For she was the embodiment of the sensation of feeling. The love Iris gave was met in kind, and she was welcomed at the gates of the underworld as readily as she was greeted in the higher realm of light. Ultimately, her inspired efforts were in service to the feminine, balancing the heart and head through her understanding of emotions and suffering. In this sense, Iris owns the rainbow—her divine expression of the multi-dimensional qualities of human consciousness and feeling.

Goethe, in his work on the theory of color, demonstrated, with the help of prisms, that the rainbow effect is not caused by a breaking up of white light, but rather by an inner weaving of light and dark elements. He, therefore, concluded that color is, itself, "the deed and suffering of light." In other words, it is, paradoxically, both the presence and the absence of light. Just as Iris, Goddess of the Rainbow, traveled through the lower and upper regions with the graceful flow of an angelic dancer, so, too, the individual on a spiritual quest must learn to journey through something very much like the rainbow (with its radiant bands of color, signifying various dimensions of experience), in order to live an art-filled life. Iris gifts humanity with the understanding that all aspects of life are sacred; and, furthermore, it is in the weaving of the dark and light within ourselves that we find our wholeness. In order to discover our true creative expression, we travel into the song of the rainbow, guided by Iris, who lovingly cloaks us with the iridescent light of our own soul.

Healing

Art is born through the soul. The healing journey of Iris offers you an ensouled vision of your flowering intuitive and feeling Self—one in which you may encounter the many hues of your emotional spectrum. We heal ourselves and others by first contacting the inner nourishment or the "water of life" which sustains our ability to create beautiful things in the world as well as to act from our hearts. Iris comes to you to awaken the ever-flowering magic and creativity that resides, like a bubbling spring, deep within you. Allow this well to be tapped into and you will experience an overflowing and abundant source of energy and inspiration. Let Iris greet you there and touch your heart and soul with her Rainbow healing. The root of your being, like the golden bulbs of the Iris, will produce the wondrous color of your potential, much like a golden chalice produces the elixir of love.

Practical Application

Iris is the paintbrush of the Soul. When we are in need of renewal through creative expression, the Iris essence serves as a chalice, or painter's cup, that can be dipped into time and again in order to paint the inner origins of our private landscape. Due to its watery signature, Iris blends the feeling world with the fiery heights of inspiration. Therefore, it is the perfect essence for artists and writers.

For example, Karen, the artist for the Power of Flower cards, used Iris essence a lot during the time she was painting the flowers. I made an essence from the Irises in my garden and gave some to her. She found my homemade essence more potent than the other Iris essences I had mixed for her. There is something very special about making essences from your own land and sharing them with the people closest to you. When Karen was exhausted and feeling low on inspiration, I would mix a combination of Elm and Iris for her, as these two flowers work very well together when one is overwhelmed and too spent to find creative motivation. We often joked about the need for gallons of Iris, for it seemed to be the elixir that would reopen the channels of creativity for us.

My daughter, Gabrielle, is a very talented young artist. During her many years at the Waldorf School, she was given the opportunity to blend a world of color and feeling. Her style is bright, deep, and full of movement. I was blessed to witness the work of Iris in a very specific way with her, and I will never forget the vivid example that Iris showed us. Gabrielle was working on a large art project for her eighth grade class. She was painting a castle, which was supposed to be rich with gardens, gates, and fantasy. At about the half way mark, the project seemed rather stressed, tight, and pale. She complained of feeling uninspired, so I prepared an Iris essence for her. The contrast between the first and second halves of the project was so astounding I saved it as a showpiece for my lectures on flower essences. The second half was rich in color and abundant with flowers and deep, green garden life. It flowed with hues of expression and a kind of magic that only the Iris could have revived within her. Without doubt, the Iris is a rainbow bridge to transformation.

For a very potent floral combination for the artist, combine Iris, Indian Paintbrush, and Blackberry. I keep a bottle of this flower bouquet in my office cabinet for those times when I am in need of a creative boost. It really works.

Iris essence can be made by the lay person very easily. If you have Irises growing in your garden, or have access to a forest floor where Wild Iris or Blue Flag grows, consider making an essence for yourself. At sunrise, when the Earth is moist, and the dew rises up through the darkness to meet the Sun, go to the Iris, attune to its beauty and radiant color, and peer inside its floral cup. Nestled inside the cave of the flower you will see tiny droplets of moisture. Collect these with a sterile dropper and put them into a dropper bottle. Fill the bottle with equal parts brandy and mineral water. Screw the lid on and tap the bottom of the bottle several times in order to wake up the essence.

Violet

LATIN: Viola Odorata

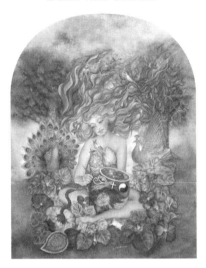

Blessing

Garden of violets is a paradise,
Where the reverence of Eve is Reborn.
With passion and self-love within me,
I embody the beauty of Earth's purity.
Within my soul, I am free.

Plant Signature

Violets are a delicate perennial flower producing long-stalked runners called stolons. The heart-shaped leaves clustered in rosettes seem to hug the earth by their close proximity to it. Sweetly scented, violets bloom from April through June. The ancient Athenians, Romans, and Celts held this plant in high regard for its various healing properties.

Flower Essence

First and foremost, the violet is a flower of modest simplicity. As an elixir, it is especially attuned to highly evolved and fragile souls—those with acute sensitivity to their surroundings as well as to other people. The violet essence help us stay true to ourselves while remaining open to our environment. It is therefore useful in the strengthening of group and individual relationships. The violet's heart-shaped leaves attract a quality of sweetness which it offers to humanity through its sweet, delicate scent. It is said to be sacred to all fairies, in particular the Fairy Queen.

Archetype
Eve

Perhaps no creation myth has been more damaging to women and the feminine principle than the story of Eve in Paradise. Held up as the embodiment of evil, we are taught to cast her out of our psyches as a way of cleansing ourselves of all that she has come to represent. We do this at our own peril, however. For in banishing Eve, we do a terrible violence to ourselves, jeopardizing our very survival as a species. Her story must, therefore, be retold (minus its patriarchal trappings), and this new story, or myth, must then be deeply implanted in the hearts and minds of humanity. In doing so, ultimately, we may achieve a true balance of masculine and feminine principles, becoming whole human and spiritual beings in the process.

Eve was once known as "Goddess of All Living Things." It is said that she wove the material of the cosmos into her various off-spring, each of whom embodied something of her inner life and purpose. The World Tree from which she allegedly ate, thereby bringing sin and death into the world according to the patriarchal story, was heralded by the ancients as a symbol of spiritual equilibrium and immortality. It was the "primal mother at the central place on Earth." Her branches reached toward the heavens, "with fruit shining like stars." This Tree of Life was considered the embodiment of the primal and abundant life force within the body of the Goddess, the Life Giver. In eating from the tree, Eve nourished herself with nature's love for her and for all humanity. The Garden of Eden, itself, represented the land of Canaan, where the Mother Goddess was honored and worshipped, before the arrival of the nomadic people who would eventually come to worship only the male God known as Yahweh.

The evil serpent, or snake, in the story of Eve in Paradise, is actually revered in many cultures as the bringer of a new stage in human evolution: self-consciousness. Similarly, the alchemical serpent held the mystery of eternity as well as of cycles of birth and death. In pre-patriarchal times, both the snake and the female body were considered sacred, for it was believed that they carried the secret of life and death.

A radical leap in consciousness must be accomplished if we are to bring Eve into the future with us. For she has been the primary scapegoat of patriarchal Western culture, vilified by his-story and sacrificed as an evil temptress. In the Hebrew text, Eve is named Isha, meaning woman. As such, she is the first woman; she is all women. In allowing Eve to individuate from the patriarchal bondage cast upon her, we can free ourselves from within of our own bondage to patriarchal myths and systems. We can truly incarnate bringing our own precious consciousness fully to bear upon the many challenges of the human condition. We can begin to honor Eve in all her primal power and goodness. The time for this type of reevaluation and reclamation is long past due.

Healing

Eve has come to you today to offer you the opportunity for true liberation at all levels. An inverted heart-shaped violet leaf, representing devotion and transcendent wisdom, covers her heart. Her hair, symbolizing the ego, is adorned with birds, symbolizing the soul, and blends naturally into the Tree of Knowledge which stands behind her. In this way, the false dichotomy between self-consciousness and spiritual growth is overcome and we begin to understand that Eve's eating the fruit of the Tree of Knowledge did not instigate a Fall into Original Sin. Rather, it introduced into the world for the first time, the real possibility of fully embracing and consciously knowing our own innate divinity.

Nature is your guide and consort, assisting you as you create the vision of a New World; one that honors difference without hardening into dualism; one that achieves a balance between the heart and mind.

In peace and tranquillity, Eve sits among the violets as the newly-hatched serpent rebirths itself. This is a time of celebration, for life's mysteries are beginning a new cycle of rejuvenation. You are invited into Eve's sacred garden. How might you weave the world as you self-liberate into the image of a New Woman? Nature surrounds you as your sister and the tender violets beckon you to enter into divine union with your Original Self.

Practical Application

The tender beauty of the Violet in the garden is a reflection of the sweet, innocent beauty of the Feminine Soul. Women of all ages and races are graced with an inner matrix of Love which is carried within the deep protection of the womb. In a world that has become overbearing and cut off from the wisdom of the Inner Feminine, many women feel fundamentally unsafe, even under siege, as they struggle to secure a positive self-image and place for themselves while honoring their womanly rhythms and sensibilities. In addition, there are women who are inherently shy and quiet, who possess a quality of refinement that may, at times, make them appear aloof or untouchable. Violet essence helps to recapture or retain the refined and tender qualities of feminine beauty, while opening to the bounty of self-expression and individuation. For these reasons, Violet is a wonderful essence to use in a woman's group.

For example, I was leading a woman's group last year and

one woman, Marianne, spoke repeatedly about feeling stifled in her marriage. She is a beautiful woman with tremendous artistic potential who had devoted much of her time and energy to raising her children. I spread the Power of Flower cards in the center of the circle, face down, and had each woman choose a card that would indicate the quality of healing coming to her. Upon receiving the Violet card, with its message of freedom and liberation, and its image of the flaming-haired Eve, so contented in Her Garden, Marianne burst into tears and cried with joy for the affirmation in her heart; the affirmation that she, too, must find that place of peace and serenity within. I gave her Violet essence to take, and several weeks later, she began to reveal an inner strength that would assist her as she liberated herself from her many ghosts of past repression. To my surprise, one very special evening, the other women in the group brought Marianne living symbols inspired by the objects depicted in the Violet card. One woman brought her Eve's apple. She also received a peacock feather, symbolizing the all-knowing wisdom within her, and a basket of fresh figs. When Marianne took a big, juicy bite of the red apple, we all gasped with delight. Eve's apple would be the first delicious fruit from the Tree of Life to nourish her inner life. She has gone on to explore her own budding individuality with grace and integrity.

I also often use Violet essence with children. This remedy, with its heart-shaped leaves, helps nourish the heart of innocence, and is useful when a child exhibits overly shy characteristics that are brought about by the stress of performance anxiety or high expectations. The purple color of the flower works delicately on the upper chakras (extending upward from the heart), aligning the child to his or her guardian angel, or Divine Love. This protection can be amplified by placing a Violet plant in the child's room with his or her picture propped against it. In addition, a spray of pure mineral water and Violet essence can be spritzed in the room for several days to enhance the quality of Violet in the child's life.

Sunflower

LATIN: Helianthus

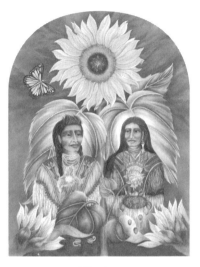

Blessing

Torch of Sunflower,
Spiral of light,
Lead me to the path of Service,
And clear insight.

Plant Signature

*T*he Greek word for Sunflower, Helianthus, literally means sun (heli) and flower (anthus). Found predominantly in North America, the Sunflower can grow to an astonishing twelve feet in height as it reaches longingly for the sun throughout the summer months. Its stem is sturdy and strong, with large leaves that are toothed at the margins. The round, flat discs at the center of its large, golden-yellow flowers are intricately composed of tiny tubular flowers arranged in a spiral design. At the end of the summer, the Sunflower's bows its mighty head toward the earth, as if in reverence to Mother Nature, offering Her its many seeds.

Flower Essence

Sunflower essence carries a radiant quality of light to the human soul, for it is associated with the sun and the conscious, enlightened self. The elixir of this flower also balances masculine and feminine archetypes. For example, as one ventures into leadership positions, Sunflower essence offers the upright, majestic power of a well-defined, masculine will, even as it opens the heart to a luminous, feminine quality of love and compassion, easing rigid patterns that create power and dominance struggles in relation to others. This essence interweaves the energy of solar fire and moist earth. Its golden light heals the solar plexus where old trauma is stored, and balances the first chakra so that one may come to rest safely in one's own power.

Archetype
THE SOLAR KING AND LUNAR QUEEN

The Sunflower towers high above the earth, reaching toward the Sun, and, ultimately, sacrificing itself in sweet surrender to cosmic service. Its spiraling roots and circular growth pattern point the way to a purification and restoration of the ego, for the Solar King's ego must be transformed by the rays of Sol, the eternal Sun. Once transformed in this way, the ego must then offer itself up to the Lunar Queen—to the face of the moon as it shimmers across a darkened world. The path of the Solar King and Lunar Queen directs us to a place of indestructible purity within—a sanctuary of true Selfhood where the Divine Will of the enlightened male combines with the Universal Love of the enlightened female. Like the Sunflower, this golden couple rises to full power by first reaching toward the light above, and then bowing to the midnight within. They reside in your heart, guiding you to whatever heights your destiny requires. The strength and integrity of this inner union will support you as you enter the realm of world service.

Healing

The Sunflower is indigenous to North America and was originally cultivated by the first known people to live on this continent, Native American Indians. The ancestors honored the cycles of nature, and in this context, worshipped the Sunflower as a symbol of the continuity of future generations and the passage of the sun through the heavens—for the flower carries within it many seeds and many cycles. Sunflower teaches you that the will to live, the will to survive, and the will to be integral, honoring Earth Mother and her bountiful resources, are essential aspects of your Earth Walk. When the Sunflower makes its appearance, she enters the garden of your life, bestowing radiant golden light, symbolizing higher vision and keen awareness. The power that is granted through Sunflower is always offered to one who is grateful and humble in their Earth Dance. This is your gift, to walk lightly upon the Earth while shouldering mighty vows of service.

Practical Application

When gazing into the mandalic mirror of a client's astrological chart, I often find that words are not enough, especially if someone is seriously suffering under the influence of a challenging transit and in the throes of a death and rebirth process. This is often when flower essence are called into play. Sunflower essence is frequently the essence of first resort during such times. For those of you who are aware of astrology, you know that the cycles of Saturn can be quite trying on an individual. When a person is seeking healing with the inner father, authority figures, in general, and/or power issues in his or her life, Sunflower is a bright torch of hope lighting the way to greater empowerment. In addition, I often prescribe Sunflower essence to clients who are, themselves, in positions of leadership and authority, especially when there is a crisis and people are questioning the power structure within the organization. It is useful when a individual has been given responsibility for a project and is feeling insecure about his or her ability and competence.

Sunflower and Larch essence, when taken together, can move one through times of deep transformation when the Self is less sure footed than usual. This combination assists in the process of becoming a true leader. It can also help with proper management of the details of one's future. When combined with Larch and Trumpet Vine, Sunflower essence can help decrease stage fright and fear of public speaking. Give Sunflower to children when you notice leadership potential in their character. This will balance the young soul, facilitate fair play and reduce the tendency to engage in power struggles.

A lovely Shaman from Mexico was visiting my city and many came to hear him speak on the topic of the cycles of the of Mayan calender. On a sunny day, on the open lands where he presented his talk, he pointed to the Sun, motioned with his hand to his heart, and said to us, "You are the Sunflowers of the earth. Walk toward the light with humility and serve the world with love. That is all there is. It is simple."

Oriental Poppy

LATIN: Paparer orientale

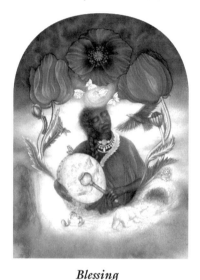

Blessing

Blazing Poppy,
Bearer of Dreams,
A Shaman's call,
To magical schemes.
Guide me into light and dark,
A path of transformation,
I embark.

Plant Signature

*T*he Oriental Poppy has brilliant orange blossoms which open dramatically, facing the sun. When fully exposed to light, the blossom's deep black centers reveal spider-like shapes within. The Poppy's rich green, fern-like leaves grow in clusters and the plant produces many large, long-stemmed bulbs resembling drumsticks. After the flower has blossomed and its petals have fallen to Earth, the dried bulbs become delicate rattles. The Poppy can withstand extreme weather conditions such as scorching sun and freezing rain. It is hardy, yet profoundly delicate by nature.

Flower Essence

The Poppy essence can have an intoxicating, uplifting effect, giving one access to the higher vibrations of the fairy world, as well as to the iridescent colors created by flower fairies. Since opium is derived from the Poppy flower, its essence is capable of bringing one into a deep state of enchantment and opening the psychic channels. This is not a drug-induced experience, however, but a very subtle and pure engagement with Nature. The Oriental Poppy essence beckons one to journey into the mysteries of creative visualization and dream journaling. Such journeys are not unlike those of ancient Shamans who traveled to the upper and lower worlds, discovering guides and animal spirits, and retrieving lost aspects of Self. This essence is an excellent remedy for those who wish to enhance their clairvoyant and telepathic skills.

Archetype
SHAMAN

Shamans are powerful healers and spiritual teachers found in indigenous cultures throughout the world. As the wise elders and medicine doctors of their tribal communities, these highly-respected men and women are intimately familiar with the hidden dimensions of Nature in all Her forms.

The Shamans' Way is a path of the heart involving profound reverence for the natural world at its deepest levels. As we descend into Her mysteries, the artificiality of such categories as "human vs. nature" and "spirit vs. matter" begins to fall away. We see that no real separation exists when one is in constant rhythm with plants, stars, animals, insects, birds, stones, and mountains, and that Nature is a sanctuary, a sacred womb, where body and soul truly meet. The Shaman guides us into the "dream body," or "shaman body," where we attune to the transformative reality of everyday miracles, seeking answers to life's most important questions.

Healing

The Poppy Shaman calls you back to your true home in Nature, where your soul speaks directly to you, delivering its many sacred messages. Deep in your heart, the muses are aroused and the plant and animal spirits surround you. Vibrant rainbow colors swirl around the Poppy Shaman's head, symbolizing the divine rays of unity and harmony that exist only when one has attuned to Nature and Her consorts in the deepest possible way. The white butterflies who bask in the translucent colors of the rainbow are signs of transformation, for the deep core of the Oriental Poppy calls you to the dark mysteries that dwell, paradoxically, within the light. The Shaman's bright orange robe shimmers with passion, stimulating the creative center that exists just below the navel. It is from this place, the womb chakra, that psychic energy is birthed. Dragonfly, polar bear, lion, eagle, fish, and caterpillar are the sacred totems of the Poppy Shaman. To which of these spirits are you most attuned?

Practical Application

This essence is very special to me. In fact, Poppy was my nickname during a very magical period in my life. Poppy was a name that seemed to offer attunement to nature's mysteries. The name Poppy saw me through my adventures in Hawaii for four years, in my late teens and early twenties, where the passion of the islands filled my heart with joy and a love for nature beyond explanation, and later through most of my stay at the Findhorn Foundation in Scotland, where the devic world became a living myth within the sanctuary of my Soul.

I began making Poppy essence several years ago, and used it during my own rituals and meditations. When I first spied an Oriental Poppy, I was in awe. This flower was enchanting and mysterious: the flame of its bright orange blossoms seemed to mirror the creative/sexual second chakra of the human body, where primordial memories are stored. I knew the Oriental Poppy wanted to be made into an essence, and that I would need to make it. Timing and syncronicity seem to govern my life in strange ways, and within two days, my neighbor brought me some cuttings to plant in my garden. The following spring season would reveal an astonishing array of Oriental Poppies, more than I had planted, plentiful and enormous.

I felt certain that the essence made from this flower could assist people on their journeys, especially shamanic journeys, into other realities and dimensions. Oriental Poppy essence has been passed around before sweat lodges, and in sacred circles, and is, in fact, used by practicing shamans. When journeying with another, it is very good to take the essence together as it enhances the etheric connection between two people. I have connected this flower with the Death card in the Tarot, for it can take us through dreams and sleep cycles, offering a glimpse into the unknown regions of our re-birth potential.

I have shared the Oriental Poppy essence with many people and have received affirmative response regarding its effectiveness. In a strange way, I feel myself to be guardian to this essence, and am honored to share it with the public through the Power of Flower cards.

Purple Water Lily

LATIN: Nymphaea

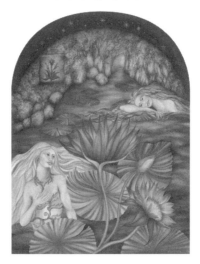

Blessing
The Water Lily nymph,
Weaves a purple web of light.
She lifts the veil of heaven,
Offering vision and sight.

Plant Signature

*T*his perennial, aquatic herb grows in streams, ponds, and marshes, as well as near the coastline. Its beautiful purple flowers rest on the surface of the water surrounded by smooth, shiny dark green leaves, and supported by a thick, horizontal root-stock below. The blossoms of the Purple Water Lily open as the sun rises, then close gradually after only a few hours, being entirely closed during the midday heat and at night. Its petals are numerous, much like the lotus, and hold a multitude of seeds within its globular fruit.

Flower Essence

The essence of the Purple Water Lily is similar to that of the Lotus, in that it is very sensitive and refined. Both also share a watery habitat, and, therefore, act as aquatic midwives to the soul, gently ushering one into the watery depths of the feeling world and assisting in the process of spiritual rebirth. This subtle yet powerful essence has the potential to bring spiritual sensitivities to the fore, drawing one inextricably into the fertile well of deepest knowing. Just as the Purple Water Lily flower closes itself to the midday heat, so must we all learn to turn the light of consciousness into the moist folds of introspection and mystery.

The elixir has a profound effect on the crown and brow chakras, opening channels of communication with vast, unseen worlds, as well as with one's own higher self. Taken before meditation or sacred ritual, it has the ability to open the portals of consciousness, guiding one into the inner sanctum of the soul, where life, death, and rebirth are unified. Just as the Purple Water Lily flower reaches toward the light of the sun, though its stem and root system remain obscured under the surface of the water, so the flower of human consciousness must reach for the light of spiritual inspiration even while our physical bodies labor under the illusions inherent in material existence. This essence not only enables the human body to absorb higher light frequencies, but also acts as a metaphor for how such a thing can be accomplished.

Archetype
WATER NYMPHS

Mythical beings of epic proportion, the Water Nymphs ignite our imagination, offering inspirational images and ineffable visions of beauty and grace. Their primary task is to overlight the particular dimension of soul-travel where the soul meets the solid world of form. They assist those who travel from one realm to the next, offering a purple garment of light to each human soul who wishes to incarnate. While holding the secrets of time and space, these spiritual mid-wives unite the lower regions of the unconsciousness—their watery, womb-like habitat—with higher aspirations and heavenly splendor—their perfected female form where sacred procreation is manifest. In serving as a bridge between the worlds, the Water Nymphs have become highly skilled at adapting to the four elements: earth (their bodies); air (their breath and wisdom); fire (their passion and regeneration); and water (their life-giving spiritual wombs). They are the Weavers of the Mysteries; their magical water a liquid crystal, repatterning the holographic potential of the universe.

Healing

The cave temples of the Water Nymphs contain two portals: one to accommodate the decent of humanity; the other to assist in the ascension of spirit. The portals face north and south, symbolizing the alchemical adage: As Above, So Below. As you attune to the subtle mysteries of the Nymph and the Purple Water Lily, you are able to transcend the limitations of linear time, and move beyond the confines of mortal existence. For her cave portals are, in fact, crystal windows of immortality, beckoning you forward on your journey of enlightenment. The Nymph's earth vessel holds the purifying waters of the soul, where a spiritual baptism or holy encounter with the elements of life can occur. Allow the watery, womb-like container to embrace and nurture you, so that you may safely hear the heavenly tones of star-filled messages which are coming your way at this time. Imagine a purple garment of light surrounding your entire body as you open the gates of new awareness. You are truly blessed to receive such an image of grace.

Practical Application

When I first heard of this essence, I knew that I needed to have it. This Lily of the water accentuates the Lily's potential to guide us down the stream of life to our inner emotions and feelings. The Lily is a feeling flower, highly tuned to subtle vibrations, and able to assist humanity in developing intuitive skills and the practice of visualization. The purple ray of the flower unites the crown chakra with the overlighting canopy of mystery represented by the starry heavens. This flower leads one through the portals of time and space. It is extremely beneficial at this time in history, when the shift in human consciousness is accelerating toward new modes of awareness.

There are stellar moments, related to the phases and aspects of the planets, when auspicious awakenings resound throughout the collective body. New dimensions of healing and universal understanding become available to us at these times. We perceive with greater subtlety than before, the fabric of life that has held us in its embrace all along. What mysterious force directs the threads through this loom of existence, we might ask?

For many, there is a longing to engage with this mystery in order to untangle the threads of illusion that tell us we are separate from each other and from the infinite. Purple Water Lily helps in this untangling.

This is another essence that I save for special events and circumstances. I offer it to friends and clients during times of great transition when they are facing serious crossroads. From the muddy depths of the soul, we search for light and warmth, the pushing up into new insights and revelations, the blossoming and triumph of the radiant Self. This is all the work of Purple Water Lily essence.

Hibiscus

LATIN: *Hibiscus rosa-sinensis*

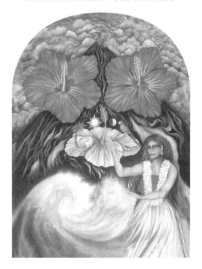

Blessing
Red Hibiscus, I greet your flame,
Hi'iaka, I call your name.
Teach me your sacred song and dance.
My soul full of passion, you enhance.

Plant Signature

*T*he hibiscus is an evergreen shrub, native to tropical Asia and subtropical regions. Found along roadsides and in uncultivated regions, as well as in show gardens and paradise parks, this hardy plant flowers all year round, with new buds appearing each morning, and red or purplish blossoms lasting only a day or two. The reproductive organs of the hibiscus flower protrude conspicuously from the center of its five flaring petals. When dried, they make an exquisite addition to your afternoon tea, bringing a warm red glow to the experience.

Flower Essence

Tropical flowers make very potent essences because they are infused with sun and rainbow colored air, both of which amplify Devic (soul) consciousness. Bursting with vitality and passion, the flaming red Hibiscus flower makes a highly charged flower remedy, indeed. It energizes the first and second chakras, undoing blockages in the lower back and spine, and healing reproductive ailments, including infertility problems. Issues concerning one's sexuality are soothed and warmed with Hibiscus essence, as well, especially in cases where frigidity or lack of feeling are obstacles to free sexual expression. Encoded with the pure innocence of female creativity and procreativity, this very feminine elixir also acts as a balm for the long held scars of sexual trauma. If you are drawn to dance as a healing modality, this essence may be particularly appropriate for you. It gets one's juices flowing, so to speak, stimulating a desire to understand bodily rhythms as well as to move one's body rhythmically. Hibiscus essence can be rubbed externally on the sacral chakra located two to three inches below the navel, in addition to being taken orally, if one wishes to enhance its therapeutic effects.

Archetype

Hi'iaka-I-ka-poli-o-Pele (Hi'iaka-in-the-bosom-of-Pele)

The mythology of the Hawaiian Goddess Pele, Goddess of Fire, is interwoven with the threads of several lovely stories, songs, and dances involving her little sister Hi'iaka. According to legend, both were born of the Earth Mother Goddess Haumea—Pele in the shape of flames; Hi'iaka as an egg that transformed into a beautiful girl. In one particularly enchanting story, Hi'iaka gathers flowers, weaves them into leis, and, through song and dance, practices the sacred, healing art of the Hula. Many of Pele and Hi'iaka's passionate adventures revolve around the dancing and singing of the Hula. In fact, so closely are the two sisters associated with this ancient practice, that Hi'iaka is considered the Supreme Goddess of the Hula, and all prayer chants and dance celebrations are said to be under her authority. It is also commonly believed that such chants and celebrations are not composed by mortals at all, but taught by the Pele spirits. Hula is a sacred study, undertaken by aspiring healers and sorcerers. In days of old, an individual was sent to the volcano in order to learn the appropriate prayers of protection and purity related to its practice. Those who mastered the art of the Hula were to offer their gifts of dance and song to Pele and Hi'iaka in a dream chant.

Healing

The Hawaiian Islands are a place of high mythological drama, with the greatest drama of all centering upon the antics of Pele and Hi'iaka, for these two legendary sisters bring the fiery passion of the volcano and the liberating sensuality of the Hula to life. Together, they bridge the mystical gap between the unseen powers of nature and humanity, for Pele is fire, itself, and Hi'iaka is the living human form of that passion. Pele can transform herself into a mortal woman, but she cannot sustain this form, for her realm is that of raw, volcanic energy. Hi'iaka becomes a living embodiment of Pele's explosive power, coupled with the qualities of compassion, service, human love and sexuality.

The Hibiscus flower comes to you today as a flaming chalice, inviting you to live your truest passions. The fires of Pele give rise to dancing flames of swirling intensity— leaping toward the heavens. Their movement serves as a metaphor, showing the way to true liberation. Hi'iaka's beautiful dance reveals the physical embodiment of Pele's fire, reminding you that you must ground this energy in your body. Swaying, undulating, and flowing to the rhythm of the cosmos strengthens the root chakra, allowing you to become rooted and safe in a world of inevitable change and uncertainty.

Perhaps most of what is wrong with the Western world can be traced to the fact that we have forgotten how to move our hips! Hibiscus thaws that which needs thawing, the frozen places inside where our passion cannot live—especially in the region of the first and second chakras. Hi'iaka gracefully moves her body to the cosmic tune of nature's symphony. Dancing amidst pounding shores and an erupting volcano wreathed in flowers and nature's garment, she creates the story of life. Choose to live your life to the flowing rhythms of the dance and bring harmony into each day. Journey to the ocean, a mountain, or your own special nature retreat in order to experience the dance of the elemental world. Feel the warmth of the inner feminine tending the hearth of your creative passion as you sip Hibiscus tea by a warm fire. Your volcanic spirit is dormant no longer. Arise and move your hips. You are alive and well.

Practical Application

When clients come to me seeking ways to open new channels of inspiration, the problem is often that they are too much in their heads, cut off from the juices of creativity flowing through their bellies and loins. Hibiscus essence is a powerful ally for the anchoring of cosmic energy. The deep red flame of this flower activates the fiery root chakra. In the alchemical process that ensues, the raw sexual and creative energy of the first chakra is infused with the energy of the soul body. Hibiscus seems to penetrate the fertile regions of the womb matrix, gently warming the cauldron of feminine magic. It revitalizes and activates the impulse to move in harmony with the storms of change, helping one to flex and bend with the unpredictable circumstances of life. For most of us, it is rarely possible to fly away to the Hawaiian Islands in order to bask in the splendor of a tropical paradise, but Hibiscus essence, in ample doses, is the next best thing.

Hibiscus essence is such a rich experience, I often like to take it mixed with hibiscus and cranberry juice. Sometimes I brew a pot of deep red Hibiscus tea, add golden honey and the essence and sip to my heart's content. Whether you drink this tea on a cool autumn evening or a luscious spring morning, I can assure you of its passionate properties.

I recently saw Sara, a client who, at age fifty-six, was making a major shift in her life, quitting a corporate job that had rewarded her for being a highly competent woman in the world of work. As her cycles began to change, she found herself moving more and more deeply into the interior mapping of her Soul. Although she had chosen this new path with great conviction and courage, she was having a difficult time really surrendering to the flow of her new life. I asked if she would like to choose a Power of Flower card in order to engage with an archetype of this "something mysterious" moving within her. Upon realizing that she had chosen the Hibiscus card, she gasped, "I just planted several Hibiscus plants in my yard!" As we delved into the perfection of this syncronicity, I summarized the Hibiscus story for her. Hibiscus is associated with Hi'iaka-l-ka-poli-o-Pele (in the bosom of Pele), Pele's sister, who allegedly introduced the Hula to the Hawaiian Islands. It is a flower that invokes movement, dance, and free flowing sensuality, especially in the region of the hips. Sara confided in me that she had always wanted to be a dancer, and, in fact, had developed a stiffness in the lower back and hip region which she believed was caused by the stress of her high pressure job.

Sara decided to begin taking the Hibiscus essence. Within one week, I received a call from her stating that she had enrolled in an African dance class, was feeling very fiery and sensual, and, I wasn't surprised to hear, was planning a retreat in Hawaii. Furthermore, she plans to connect with the Hibiscus flower personally for she feels it has invited her into the passionate dance of her future. This story illustrates beautifully that even when we are not consciously aware of it, unconsciously we are creating our own magic each and every moment. Planting the Hibiscus was Sara's soul's way of setting the intention to become alive and whole again. It is not the work of the flower alone that heals the soul, but the work of our own will and love, as well.

Manzanita

LATIN: *Arctostaphyos manzanita*

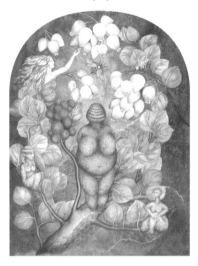

Blessing
Manzanita offers the wisdom of Goddess lore,
The beautiful roots of Her ancient core.
My body sings as I dance Her truth,
My body is beautiful in age and youth.

Plant Signature

*A*n evergreen plant, ranging in size from a creeper to a full-sized shrub, to a small, rounded tree, the Manzanita is admired for the beauty of its crooked branches which are smooth, shapely and of a deep, reddish purple color—attracting a multitude of birds. Its leaves are broad and oval in shape, and adorn the branches with a shiny, silvery green. The common Manzanita has white to pink bell-like flowers and tiny fruit resembling apples, which turn from white to a deep red.

Flower Essence

The Manzanita, with its rounded curves and dancing, bending branches, seems to embody the Goddess within her very core. It is, not surprising, then, that the tree produces tiny apple-like fruits—an ancient symbol of fertility and sensuality. Its bell-shaped flowers serve as nature's instruments, proclaiming the glory of the female form in its many shapes and sizes.

Manzanita elixir helps uplift a woman's (or man's) attitude concerning body image, in a culture that fails to honor the many varieties of the female form—inviting the Goddess in each of us to be revealed in all her splendor. This is especially important today as we embark upon a new Millennium and the immanent revival of the sacred feminine. In a world where, sadly, most women feel inadequate or even disgusted by their physical appearance, Manzanita is a much needed remedy. Nothing less than the evolution of human consciousness is at stake, for the degradation of the feminine in Her various guises is its most significant stumbling block.

This is also an excellent essence for people who suffer from eating disorders of any kind, as well as for those sensitive souls who find the physical form unpleasant—in particular, spiritually-attuned individuals who find the body cumbersome. Manzanita brings harmony to body and soul, increasing one's ability to experience the body as a beloved temple of the spirit.

Archetype

THE FERTILITY GODDESS, VENUS OF WILLENDORF

An abundance of archaeological evidence, dating from the Paleolithic and Neolithic periods, strongly suggests that ancient civilizations honored and revered the Goddess as the embodiment of sacred cycles of life and death. Her emblem of fertility, a full, round body, pregnant with the possibility of new life and creativity, was the hallmark of ancient matriarchal societies—a timeless, symbolic representation of the Universal Mother Goddess.

The Venus of Willendorf, c.2300 BCE, is a Paleolithic Venus depicted without benefit of a male consort, for it is likely that the people who lived during this ancient time in human development were unaware of the male role in procreation. In fact, they may have thought females capable of partheno-genesis, or self-impregnation. Such was the astonishing power of the Goddess, along with her Earthly counterparts.

Like the Manzanita tree, prehistoric people lived close to the Earth, and just as we admire the plants graceful curves and rounded form, the ancients loved the Goddess whose body was a shrine of productivity and beauty. To them, She was the cosmic parent who created life and exerted her considerable divine influence over the natural order of things. One would not think to defile Her, for she was procreatress—and life, itself, depended upon Her.

Healing

The Venus of Willendorf and the dancing Goddess figures in the Manzanita tree greet you, honoring the feminine spirit that resides with you. You are being mirrored by the Universal Mother who asks that you see yourself as she sees you—as an incarnation of divinity. Perhaps you need to tap your roots a bit closer to the Earth in order that you may fully take pleasure in your glorious body. As your body cycles through its many seasons, contemplate the Manzanita as a symbol of feminine transformation: its bark peels from its lovely branches after its ripened fruit has fallen to Earth, and like the snake, it then begins a new cycle of rejuvenation. The female body is nature's treasure, for without Her many symbolic deaths and regenerations, humanity would surely perish. We must once again learn to respect our female bodies, nourish them well, and love them fully, if we are to honor the Great Goddess who gives Her abundant Love to all.

Practical Application

One of the most tragic maladies afflicting our culture is the desecration of women's bodies. We project distorted and damaging images of women in the popular media, as well as through pornography, and many women have become dangerously disconnected from their natural bodily rhythms and processes while trying to match some ideal that has little or nothing to do with real women's lives. Eating disorders abound and the epidemic has begun to filter into the male population as well. The problem seems so deeply rooted in the collective feminine psyche that it is difficult to know how to approach the healing process. Manzanita essence is very useful as a remedy for women and men who have learned to relate to their bodies as objects of disgust and aversion.

Countless women have sat in my office sharing the same crisis that we all share as females: not feeling beautiful enough, good enough, worthy enough. I keep lots of Manzanita essence on hand for such clients and also stock ready made bottles when I travel. Manzanita is a sister/mother/goddess remedy, so I use it often when I lead women circles. Under the healing influence of Manzanita, women begin to appreciate the natural curves of their own sweet bodies, and seek to honor the fertile beauty in all women, without feeling envious or competitive. It can be beautifully blended with Pomegranate essence for a nurturing dose of self- assurance and empowerment.

Eating disorders of various kinds run in my family, so I have had a lot of personal experience with Manzanita and am most grateful for its healing powers. For several years a Manzanita branch hung over my bed and I would dangle little gifts and treasures to myself from it. A beautiful store in Redding, California where I led a workshop had Manzanita branches hanging off the ceiling adorned with sweet twinkling lights. I felt so nurtured and blessed in that space, and experienced the branches reverently reaching out to greet and protect each woman as she entered the store.

Bleeding Heart

LATIN: Dicentra formosa

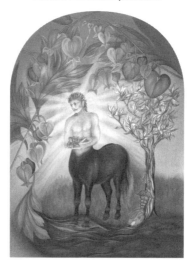

Blessing
Bleeding Heart
Expand my soul,
That I may truly see
How the journey into my suffering
Is the path to set me free.

Plant Signature

*B*leeding Heart, so named because its blossoms are perfectly heart-shaped, is native to the moist woods along the Pacific coastline. Its gentle pink or deep rose colored blooms hang in delicate clusters from a leafless red flower stalk, giving the appearance of a love offering from the Goddess. As the flower matures, it breaks open and the bottom point of each heart turns a bit upward, reminding us that "a broken heart is an open heart." Never fear, love is never lost.

Flower Essence

Bleeding Heart essence purifies and strengthens the heart chakra as well as all emotions concerning love. To those who may have closed their hearts due to fear, abandonment, or loss—especially the death of a relationship or loved one—it brings an open-hearted attitude, soothing the emotions so that one may reinvite the spirit of love into one's soul body. We are reminded, by the gentle workings of this elixir, that there is no shortage of love—that, in fact, love is showered upon us eternally by the Beloved. It is also revealed to us that the inner domain of the human heart is our most precious gift and that, ultimately, love heals all conflicts. This powerful remedy offers its unconditional love to the wounded healer in all of us. As we embrace our own suffering with tenderness, we come to understand it as a treasures of the heart which can lead us to greater awareness, empathy, and compassion for all who suffer.

Archetype
CHIRON, THE WOUNDED HEALER

Chiron is a newly-discovered planet sighted in 1977 by Charles T. Kowal of the Hale Observatory in Pasadena, California. Found "wandering" between Saturn and Uranus, this astronomical mystery is a powerful addition to the field of astrological interpretation. Named after the Centaur in Greek mythology, Chiron is thought to embody the archetypal energy of the Wounded Healer. His myth lies at the very core of human evolution for it points to our central purpose on Earth: the quest to fulfill our individual and collective destinies by courageously pursuing the "Path of the Heart." In the process of rooting our lives more and more deeply in the soil of Eternal and Unconditional Love, we heal the Wounded Healer in us all.

In Greek mythology, Chiron is the son of Cronus (Saturn) and the nymph Philyra. As the story goes, Philyra changed herself into a mare to escape Chronus' unwanted advances, but he outsmarted her by changing himself into a horse and, thereby, succeeded in mating with her. This unloving union produced Chiron who was born with the body and legs of a horse and the torso and arms of a man. In her horror and grief, upon seeing her son for the first time, Philyra pleaded with the Gods to transform her into anything other than what she was. The Gods complied with her request, turning her into a Linden tree. Thus, Chiron was abandoned later to be found by Apollo, the Sun God, who became his foster father and taught him the ways of the Healer, artist and scholar.

Through an understanding of this powerful myth, humanity may learn to heal its issues of abandonment—whether in relation to God, our parents, our life's work, or love. Apollo represents the conscious path of service. As we dedicate ourselves to the fulfillment of our destinies, we discover that we are never alone. On the Solar Heart Path, Love and Conscious Will are the greatest parents of all. Our wounds become the juice of our existence, leading us upward and onward toward the luminous Heart of God. From such a place of Eternal Peace, we come to serve the world.

Healing

Bleeding Heart opens you to the glowing warmth of the heart. This is the power of the world soul which feeds the inner fire of love and compassion. Cosmic rays of loving radiance pour through the Bleeding Heart Blossoms directly into your heart. In this way, therapeutic channels are opened and the suffering you have carried on your human journey can be healed.

Like Chiron, you have become conscious of your destiny. Sitting amongst the flowers, the centaur plays his instrument, refining the notes and tones of his inner harmonies. The Linden tree, representing Philyra, overlights him, offering support and protection as he seeks to learn the ways of nature.

Chiron has an important message for you. He offers assurance that you, too, are a healer, and that if you are to walk the path of consciousness, you must go beyond your wounds and accept this golden opportunity to metamorphose into a new body of light. The Bleeding Heart flowers bless and honor you, for your heart has been granted a new birth of consciousness which carries the seed of an emerging cosmology of health and well-being.

Practical Application

The symbol of Sufism is a heart with wings, symbolizing the unconditional forces of freedom and love. The Bleeding Heart flower resembles the Sufi symbol, for the bottom tip of this heart-shaped flower, when fully mature, splits open, unfurling wings of joy which point upward toward the light. Many of us have learned the hard way, which is perhaps the only way, that a broken heart is an open heart. Once our hearts have been truly and radically broken open, we are able to take flight, approaching our own suffering, as well as that of others, with true empathy, compassion and insight.

I could write an entire book on Bleeding Heart essence. This little gem of nature has soothed and healed so many of my clients, and myself, as well, that I feel I must bow to it in reverent gratitude whenever I come upon it, nestled in the shade, on nature hikes. Many clients, facing divorce, the death of a loved one, or even just the death of various deeply held illusions, report a feeling of tightness in the solar plexus or third chakra, the energy center in the body between the heart and belly button. So deep is their distress, that often times they cannot rest or get enough sleep. A friend or therapist may even have suggested anti-depressant medication. Sometimes this extreme measure is needed, but more often than not, Bleeding Heart essence takes the edge off one's depression to the extent that one is able to uncover new perspectives on his or her situation without the need for mood altering drugs. With the help of this gentle miracle worker, people usually report an immediate sense of the overlighting protection of Love and, consequently, much relief. I went through many bottles of Bleeding Heart, myself, during a very painful relationship break-up, and so can attest to its healing properties through firsthand experience. You know the saying "Never leave home without it." In the case of Bleeding Heart essence, I would suggest you "Never leave a relationship without it."

Often Bleeding Heart is the essence of choice when it seems nothing can help. The individual is so distraught that a flower essence consultation is just about the last thing he or she is interested in doing. This is when I make house calls. A little bottle left in a mailbox, a simple note, and a gentle suggestion that the poor suffering soul try a few drops is all I do. I might as well sit by my phone. Usually it rings within twenty-four hours, with a much lighter sounding friend or client on the other end stating in disbelief, "Gee, I don't know why but I feel much better and able to cope." Bleeding Heart, mixed with Angelica, is an especially potent combination. Angelica anchors and grounds one with the protection of Higher Forces while Bleeding Heart opens the heart to healing.

All essences work very well with animals. Bleeding Heart is excellent for a pet who has lost a beloved companion, whether of the four-footed or human variety. Our animals grieve, too. I gave Bleeding Heart to my parakeet when her partner was found dead at the bottom of her bird cage one winter morning. She hardly had the strength to stay balanced on her perch. I put one drop of Bleeding Heart in her water, and within two days, she was chirping again. This is a wonderful essence for children or adults who have to say good bye to a beloved pet.

Lavender

LATIN: Lavandula officinalis

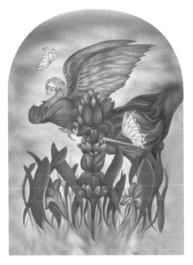

Blessing
In blessed purity,
Lavender heals,
I am protected by your immunity.
Your elixir of love protects the Earth,
Offering a salve of peace and mirth.

Plant Signature
*N*ative to Persia and Southern France, the Wild Lavender thrives where few other plants survive: on rocky barren soil at altitudes as high as 6,000 feet. Intense heat cannot harm it, nor can the bitter cold. Each year this relatively diminutive plant extends its new growth upward toward the heavens, with stems upright and vertical. Its

brilliant bluish/purple blossoms, nestled among linear, blue green leaves, become tubular at the end of he stem. Both leaves and flowers are fragrant.

Flower Essence

The botanical name Lavandula comes from the Latin lavare, meaning "to wash". The pure, clean aroma of the Lavender blossom washes one's energetic field, lending an aura of innocence and purity to all it touches. For this reason, it has long been revered by mystics, saints, and botanists the world over. For example, the medieval Christian mystic Hildegaard of Bingen is known to have recommended Lavender for the maintenance of "pure character."

As a flower remedy, Lavender soothes and heals a shattered soul force when mental and spiritual properties have become overly burdened by the demands of a "high energy" life. This bracing elixir also helps one undo negative self-talk. Thinking is infused with the quality of spiritual clarity—undaunted by the afflictions of the mind and the muddying realities of the physical world. It is as if one has breathed in the sharp fragrance of fresh, tangy mountain air. The bluish/purple vibration associated with this essence activates the throat and crown chakra, offering a sweet halo of Lavender around the head and shoulders. To fully embrace the power of this plant's healing beauty, I recommend the use of Lavender essential oil, an equally powerful therapeutic tool, in conjunction with the flower elixir.

Archetype
ARCHANGEL RAPHAEL

Pure beauty is omnipresent, yet one must reach toward the heavenly spheres in order to see and recognize it. All plants and flowers are a divine mirror of this essential truth, each flower a mini representation of angelic consciousness. Archangel Raphael, whose name literally means "God Heals" or "God Has Healed," protects and overlights the Nature Kingdom—his healing presence extending outward to envelope all Earthly beings, including plants, trees, animals, insects, rocks, and minerals, as well as humans. Through him the Earth becomes a suitable abode for humanity. Clothed in soft greens and all shades of lavender, he carries a golden vial of Lavender oil and an arrow symbolizing the stem of the Lavender plant, with arrowhead-like blossoms flowering at its tip. Raphael is focused; His intention is to heal.

Healing

The Guardian of Treasures comes to you carrying a golden potion of Lavender healing. You are under the protection of Archangel Raphael; your mental anguish and cumbersome worries are washed clean; earthly burdens are lifted; and vision is purified. You can rest peacefully. Raphael drapes His violet blue wings around you, reminding you that you are never alone on your healing journey. The white butterflies in this card represent purity and freedom, for once the mind has been cleansed, it becomes like a butterfly spreading its wings, receptive to sublime messages of liberation. If you are in need of deep healing at this time, Lavender flower elixir will soothe your soul. It is beneficial to rub the oil made from the Lavender plant directly onto your body, absorbing its healing fragrance, as well as its healing essence during times of stress, crisis, or illness. Dried lavender is also glorious; sprinkle some around your altar or meditation site, as this will invite the presence of your healing angel, Raphael.

Practical Application

The many uses and healing modalities of Lavender make it a very versatile plant. I have recommended Lavender for clients who are highly stressed and unable to slow down. Mixed with Aloe Vera flower essence, it soothes the burned out feeling and restores balance within the body so that one can begin to get some rest. I often ask such clients to attune to the purple flame of passion that resides within the creative center at the base of the spine. This flame allows constant, steady, and focused creativity to flow through the body, accessing the energy called kundalini, which awakens the life force.

Lavender essence has also been very useful for people who have back problems and are feeling stiff in the spine. I recommend it for people who are just beginning a yoga class or some other form of stretching and rejuvenating body movement.

I live in a university town so it is not unusual to see clients who are pursuing doctoral or master's degrees. They often call when deadlines are hitting, and the stress of study is becoming too much to handle. I typically prescribe Lavender essence at such times, as it soothes the spine, which in turn, relaxes the shoulder and head area. It can be a great remedy to take before exams or high pressured interviews. The calming effect of the Lavender does not disturb the mental faculties. Instead, one is simultaneously alert and at ease. By the time stress has accumulated to the point of invading the bodies immune system it is difficult to get back on track without some rebalancing through vibrational remedies, massage, or other modes of healing. This is when Lavender can be the greatest aid.

Buttercup

LATIN: Raminculus bulbosus

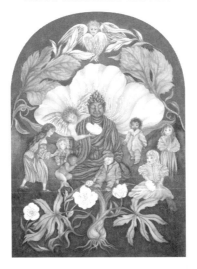

Blessing
Oh, Buddha Buttercup,
Your Sunshine Love bathes me
With golden light.
Innocence is restored,
My True Self shines bright.

Plant Signature

*A*lso known as Goldcup, the Buttercup is a dazzling yellow flower covering Spring meadows with vibrant color. Though not technically a member of the bulb species, the plant is bulb-like in nature. Due to the nourishment stored in its bulb, the Buttercup blooms prolifically and is one of the first flowers to herald the beginning of Spring. Its petals are soft and buttery, and somewhat shiny, like the sweet skin of a baby. Its upper leaves are long, narrow segments; while the lower ones are more broadly cut into distinctive masses.

Flower Essence

The translucent yellow light emanating from the Buttercup blossom transmits a tender message of love to humanity. Its essence carries a blessing of quiet surrender, beckoning one to "ride the magic carpet" of blissful love into the inner regions of the Essential Self, where purity and innocence reside. Here one is infused with the infinite, the eternal, the luminous. This is a beautiful remedy for children and adults, alike, who yearn for the sacrament of their angelic essence, their "original face before they were born." Buttercup restores and heals the inner child, helping us remember the creative gifts we carry into this world, for the spirit of the sacred child arises within the human heart when this remedy is taken.

Archetype
DIVINE CHILD

For many adults, the purity and bliss of the "radiant child within" is long forgotten—a mere figment of the imagination. Sadly, many have lost sight of the spiritual essence of love that once pervaded their souls, for in the process of "growing up," they have lost contact with the magical realm which is the soul of the child. At last, we collectively begin to hear the cry of this genius Child Self who holds the key to enlightened creativity, understanding that all such activity is ultimately divine play. Deep in the caverns of the Self, a beautiful aspect of tenderness lives, waiting for the awakened moment when it may join in life's sweet journey into love.

Healing

The Divine Child, known in Tibetan Buddhism as the Child Luminosity, will never abandon you; instead, the child waits patiently for a time of reunion with the Mother Luminosity, or pure consciousness. In this way, the heart of the child meets the wisdom inherent in all of Life. This integration of Divine Mother and Child is essential as you embark on the healing quest of Self Love and maturation. The process of discovering the golden cup of love within is nothing short of enlightening, for the holiest of holies resides in the Buttercup meadow of your heart.

Just as the child angel in this card holds a Buttercup over the heart of the Buddha, so too is your heart being offered a precious gift of Nature. It is time to accept the luminous child which is your birthright, and to hold dear the treasure of your Originally Enlightened Self. The Buttercup behind the Buddha reflects an aura of golden light, symbolizing your own Luminous Child Self which guides you at all times. Its radiant light penetrates your solar body, or solar plexus—the area below your heart where emotion and feeling are stored. The Buttercup's enlightened energy field bestows many blessings upon you and offers you clarity, so that you may see the Truth of who you really are.

Practical Application

In addition to treating adults with flower essences, I have also had the good fortune to work with children. Flower essences and children make a perfect match, for the child mind is wide open to the vibrations of flower spirits and nature's angels. When working with a child, I like to speak to them about the flowers as dear helpers and friends who lend their color, beauty, and bounty to us like rainbows in the garden. When in need of peace and comfort, we can go to the rainbow carpet of the flower world, and choose a flower that wants to help us at that particular time. Conversely, we can aid the flowers by admiring them as we walk past, and by stopping to experience the scent of their delicate blossoms. Flowers love us so much, it is sad that we do not love ourselves in return.

Buttercup, the little golden chalice of the meadow, adores children and the child within us all. It offers us its golden light so that we may shine forth, mirroring its sweet innocence. Buttercup essence is perfect for children who are experiencing low self-esteem and unable to appreciate the creative gifts that are their own unique contributions to the world. Buttercup generally brings the rosy shine of contentment back into a little one's cheeks. If a child has been teased or hurt, Buttercup can remind her that she is still loved and cherished.

I had the good fortune of coaching my daughters' softball team many years back. For three successive years I worked with these girls, often administering flower essence before, during, and after a game. They all especially loved Buttercup essence, and would line up like little birdies in a nest, tongues held out in anticipation, as I dispensed the night's supply of Buttercup essence, while puzzled onlookers wondered just exactly what it was we were doing. It was a sight I will never forget. Buttercup seemed to allow each girl the opportunity to display her own special gifts while admiring and honoring her other team members, and even members of the other team. We had one of the most harmonious teams in the league and were often complimented for our outstanding sportsmanship.

When I do my Inner Child workshops with the Inner Child Cards, I use Buttercup as the main essence for the group. It mysteriously allows access to the Divine Child within, that magical part of each of us that is pure creativity personified. When seeking contact with your own self-worth, especially if your self-worth was damaged in childhood, Buttercup is the flower of choice.

Passion Flower

LATIN: *Passiflora incarnata*

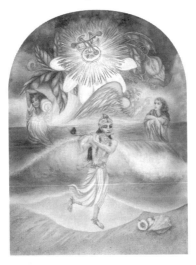

Blessing
Holy flower of the vine,
Passion Flower you are thine,
Rise above to star-light Sun,
Showering compassion on everyone.

Plant Signature

In the 16th century, Spanish explorers were enchanted by the exotic beauty of the glorious climbing vines of the Passion Flower. Named for its resemblance to the finely-cut corona at the center of Christ's Crown of Thorns, the Passion Flower's delicate flowers were thought to symbolize elements of the crucifixion: the three stigmas, which receive the pollen, representing the nails piercing the Saviors hands and feet; the five stamen representing his wounds. Some even claimed to see the cross itself in the flower's center. The vines of the plant reach to the tops of trees where their blossoms commune with the sun, in a manner reminiscent of Christ's return to the light of God through his resurrection. The sweet scented blooms of the Passion Flower are flesh-colored or yellowish and tinged with purple. Nestled in their midst is a ripe, orange colored ovoid containing hundreds of black seeds, each with a delicious, fruity interior.

Flower Passion

The Passion Flower essence anoints the soul with the "com-Passion" of Cristos, "The Anointed One" who has come to Self-Realization or Christ Consciousness through initiation into the mystery teachings. It also reawakens ancient memories of the wisdom held by Holy Orders such as the Essenes, who inhabited the Holy Land at the time of Christ. These submerged traditions carried the mystical knowledge that God, the Goddess, and Love are One, and, furthermore, that such Infinite Love exceeds all boundaries of human or material form.

This penetrating elixir helps us understand the deepest possible meaning of our own personal suffering, after which it assists in the ascent to our truest calling of service on the planet. As we truly surrender to the sorrows and hardships that have been endured in this lifetime, we begin to experience them as stepping stones or teachings that can lead to greater Love and Compassion. Passion Flower essence serves as a "bridge of light" to the human soul, helping the individual release past trauma by discovering its deeper meaning so that he or she may be resurrected into the passion and joy of life.

A literal rising up or swirling sensation can be experienced when taking this elixir, for it seeks to purify the kundalini forces which coil upward around the spine. While strengthening one's connection to Selfless Service and

Unconditional Love, it also draws one closer to angelic messengers and galactical star patterns.

Archetype
CHRISTOS, KRISHNA

The word avatar literally means "down coming," and, historically, an Avatar is understood as an incarnate Master who has graced the Earth with his presence in order to serve humanity with infinite compassion and selfless surrender. Krishna and Jesus were two such exalted beings: Krishna, considered an incarnation of Shiva, the oldest known deity in the East; and Jesus, regarded as the Holy Son of God, who embodied the Light of Solar Consciousness.

It is, perhaps, not surprising that we should find a great deal of correlation in the mystical and mythical teachings concerning Jesus and Krishna, since there is ample evidence to suggest that around the time of Christ, and even before his arrival on the world scene, a lively trade route existed between India and the Middle East. There was also extensive intermingling of these two centers of religious life, East and West. According to the legends of their respective cultures, both Jesus and Krishna were born of sacred female divinity, their forthcoming births announced to the world by a brilliant star. Both were hailed as Redeemers and World Saviors, who had descended to Earth in order to refine and attune the masses to the principle of heart-centered truth. Both were also given the higher status of God-Man or Deity, and their messages closely resembled those of World teachers and God Men who had proceeded them. Both carried the seed of Self-Knowledge from the starry regions of the heavens, implanting it in the minds and hearts of humanity. Both continue to serve as mirrors to humanity, representing the unconditional love inherent in all beings. Their truest mission is to reflect the latent divinity locked within each mortal being, serving as a living mediator between Heaven and Earth, so that the continuing passion of the soul can be understood and realized.

Healing

When Passion Flower comes to you, you are called to the inner sanctuary of your soul in order to resurrect the Divine Love and Compassion held therein. Like the vine of the Passion Flower, you reach ever upward, through whatever suffering and hardship you have experienced on your long journey, to the source of all light, which is true Self-Knowledge. While Krishna plays his magical flute, sounding the divine chords and notes of the heavens, a wave of eternity breaks behind him, and an angel, wrapped in Passion Flower wings, brings a message of Divine conception to the initiate. You are being shown your own soul's journey at this time, for you come from the stars of heaven to this earthly abode.

Satya Sai Baba, a modern day Avatar living in Puttaparti India, is, like the Avatars of old, an embodiment of Divine Love. The woman holding a jug of water represents His Holiness, for his mother was said to have received the light of a star-burst or illumination as she gathered water just prior to his conception. Once again you are given a symbol of your sacred origins, for we are all holographic images of the same Divine Reality. Like Krishna and Christ before him, Satya Sai Baba knows the true meaning of I Am Consciousness. He asks that we all recite the following prayer many times a day: "I Am God, I Am Not Separate From God. Remember who you are. Blessings."

Practical Application

The tropical flowers, infused with the moisture of the fertile earth and the warmth of the radiant sun, are in a class of their own. Just as desert flowers embody a unique attunement to the extreme environmental conditions within which they thrive, so do the flowers that grow in tropical climates.

Passion Flower is a climbing vine, always reaching higher and higher toward the light in order to find that ultimate place for blossoming, that ultimate place of rest. Are we so different from that? The developmental path of the Passion Flower is a beautiful metaphor for the quest of the human spirit, to be growing ever upward toward the light of truth, love, ultimate meaning.

Passion Flower essence has extraordinary properties. This essence reminds us that we are, in fact, living embodiments of the divine, and that for this great gift we are most fortunate. It helps us feel gratitude, and rightly so, for this precious human birth. In addition, Passion Flower overlights humanity with utmost tenderness and compassion, helping us trust that our life cycles and difficult transitions will, if fully surrendered to, eventually yield much truth, beauty and piece of mind. In this context, we are able to see our trials and tribulations as little stepping stones along the road to higher consciousness. Perhaps, at some point in our evolution we will no longer need the experience of pain and suffering in order to open our hearts and become more loving, but for now, this is one of the ways in which we can learn.

I have given Passion Flower essence to clients when they feel crucified, victimized or overly burdened by karmic situations in which they find themselves. This essence has brought great peace to many, and I often offer it with a prayer or quote from an inspirational teacher. I recommend taking Passion Flower in tandem with an attitude of thoughtful devotion and gratitude to the beings of love who oversee our path.

Silver Sword

LATIN: Argyroxiphium macrocephalum

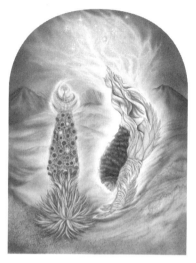

Blessing
Celestial greetings
Silver Sword brings.
Within its mystery
A Galactic tone rings.
Arise and Awaken
As the universe sings.

Plant Signature

The magnificent Silver Sword grows exclusively on the Islands of Hawaii. There are five distinct varieties of Argyroxiphium, the most famous being the Haleakala Silver Sword. It blooms among the clouds on the high slopes of Haleakala Crater in a decidedly other-worldly, moon-like environment. The plant grows in a rotund cluster of silvery, curved, spiky leaves. It remains in this configuration for over a decade, after which, a spectacular stalk of reddish-purplish florets emerges from its core, growing to a height of three to six feet. Once this one dramatic flowering is accomplished, the Silver Sword plant dies.

The roots of the Silver Sword barely penetrate the earth, making it a frequent casualty of careless humans, roving animals, and even windy weather conditions. For this reason, the plant in its undisturbed state is a rare and amazing specimen. Furthermore, given such a delicate root system, it is difficult to imagine how the relatively few plants that somehow, miraculously manage to survive are able to support the mighty stalks they eventually produce. It is as if, by the magnetic force of the heavens alone, these strange but wonderful plants are sustained in their majestic, vertical postures, reaching ever upward toward their true, celestial home. Not surprisingly, the Silver Sword is considered a distant relative of the Sunflower, another tall, gangly plant that reaches for the sky. Plentiful in the late 1800's—when Silver Swords covered the slopes of Haleakala Crater like silver snow—the plant's population declined steadily in the 1900's. Fortunately, this most unusual plant is now being carefully monitored in order to prevent its extinction.

Flower Essence

Essences from the tropical islands tend to be more refined, in general, and, must, therefore, be handled with care in order to sustain their healing properties. The Silver Sword elixir, in particular, is very rare, with a high vibratory frequency and relatively short shelf-life. It works its special brand of magic by releasing encoded information that has been stored in the miasmas, or cellular memory bank, completely opening one's energy centers and aligning one's body with the next seven chakras above the crown. Its reddish/purple flowers connect the first and seventh chakra, exposing the human body to higher frequencies of experience and strengthening the mind. The Silver Sword, with its sword-shaped leaves, serves as a harbinger of truth. Its essence cuts through the veil of illusion characteristic of ordinary reality, thereby, increasing the overall intelligence of humanity. This remedy must not be over-used, and is best taken by itself.

Archetype
CELESTIAL LIGHT-BEARER

In conventional terms, we humans are thought to be limited in our perceptions of reality by our five senses, which give us the capacity to hear, taste, smell, see, and touch—though within a very narrow range of experience. In this context, we relate to a physical environment which is made up of four general elements: earth, air, fire, and water. In the mystical, alchemical view, however, a sixth sense organ and a fifth element take us beyond our physical limitations—which are, ultimately, self-imposed anyway—into dimensions of reality where conventional wisdom no longer applies. With our sixth sense, that which intuits, has visions, and creates miracles, we are able to relate directly to the fifth element of clarity and invisible forces of light.

In many esoteric disciplines, it is taught that certain plant and mineral substances were brought to the Earth from other galaxies, planets, or stars, and that these life forms stand poised to aid and enhance the development of humanity—to take us beyond what we currently think is possible. The Silver Sword, a most unusual, other-worldly plant species, may be one such gift—brought to Earth from some other dimension for our spiritual edification. In support of this theory, many sightings of extra-terrestrial aircraft have been reported near Haleakala Crater, as it is a high energy spot of exceptional quality. When one quietly contemplates the reality of this plant, with its very delicate root system and great height, it seems entirely possible that the Silver Sword was gently and intentionally placed upon the Earth by beings from above.

If we open our hearts to possibilities beyond the material, we may become acquainted with celestial guides who overlight our journey and help us pierce the veil of illusion so that we may come to know the essential elements of our existence. These Light Bearers may not actually have a shape—perhaps they are pure energy vehicles free of the forms we attach to here on Earth. Many people who allow such higher inspiration into their lives become the greatest visionaries and geniuses of an era. Rare plants, celestial music, exquisite art, and intuitive senses—are but a few of the divine gifts humans have been given to uplift the soul and advance the evolutionary process. In the truest sense, each of us may indeed become a bearer of light in our own right.

Healing

The presence of the Silver Sword card is a rare gift. You have a heightened sensitivity and are, indeed, opening to new levels of awareness at this time. The luminous colors emanating from the Light Bearer's hands and above the Silver Sword flowers are waves of vibratory healing available to you at this time. Archetypically, the presence of this beautiful being indicates that you are bringing special gifts to the Earth through your Divine Love and Intelligence. Yoga and breathing exercises would be beneficial to you now. Sit with your back straight and aligned, allowing the energies to move freely.

Practical Application

The Silver Sword is a most rare and sacred of plants, growing solely on the summit of the Halaakea Crater in Maui. It carries the high vibration of an island flower, emphasizing the fire essence of purification and spiritual awakening, so it must be used with the greatest of care and consideration. An aligning flower, Silver Sword should be reserved for use during meditation, spiritual treks, retreats, and in some cases, when attempting to converse with other realms of consciousness, for it serves as a shimmering chord that connects us to the starry galaxies. As you can imagine, this essence is very beautiful to take when in Hawaii, especially Maui, and anyone would be most fortunate to be on the crater when the Silver Sword is in bloom. It is important to respect the request to stay away from the blossoms, but I can assure you, you can feel the radiance of these flowers from a great distance.

Upon finishing the Inner Child Cards, a Tarot deck I authored in 1993 that connects the images of fairy tales and the mythology of nature with the ancient wisdom of Tarot, I knew I wanted to initiate the deck before sending it off to the publisher. I, therefore, took a rough copy of the cards with me to the top of Haleakea Crater hoping to sit near a Silver Sword, so that I might offer the gift of clarity to the cards. When I arrived at the top of the crater at sunrise, I was amazed to find the Silver Swords in full bloom. The flowers were roped off so as not to be disturbed, so I asked the park ranger if I could go behind the rope, and, miraculously, got permission to spend some time with this most awe-inspiring of flowers. I spread my inner child cards around one especially powerful plant, and sat in reverence, visualizing the deck and book in the world as a tool for human advancement. I then asked that one card reveal the essence of the experience, and after much concentration and prayer, I chose, to my joy and amazement, the Ace of Swords. This card signified to me the deep connection I had made with the Silver Sword, and indeed, offered clarity of thought, word, and deed. An ace in the Tarot is always a blessing and a gift of new beginnings. I felt very grateful to the Silver Sword and whenever I am seeking higher attunement, I go to this flower.

I give Silver Sword to clients who seem unable to stand upright and connect with their High Self or Truth. I do not blend this essence with other essences, just as I rarely blend Lotus with anything else. These two flowers seem most potent on their own.

Shooting Star

LATIN: Dodeatheon hendersonii

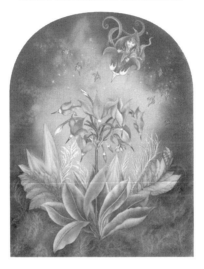

Blessing
Shooting Star expands my role,
So I may truly unite,
With the memory of my star-bright soul,
And my mission of cosmic light.

Plant Signature

S hooting Star is a spring flower. Its pale, green leaves, in delicate basal rosettes, cannot endure the summer heat. This rare plant is not adaptable to a great range of conditions. It can be found, if one is lucky, growing in meadows and other wild areas where the soil is rich and fertile and there is an abundance of water.

Shooting Star blossoms cluster on a leafless stem, reaching as much as two feet in length. Colors vary according to the species, ranging from white to pink, lavender or magenta. This beautiful little flower resembles a star or comet zooming to earth—hence, its name. The seeds of this cosmic messenger are usually not available in nurseries, so it becomes necessary to acquire them from a seed specialist or from the wild plants, themselves.

Flower Essence

As a flower elixir, Shooting Star is most beneficial to those who feel alienated from numerous aspects of earthly existence—and suffer deeply for it. They may feel an inordinate connection to plant spirits and flower elementals and/or to extraterrestrial and galactical dimensions of reality. Many were the so-called "black sheep" of their families, and report a decided lack of affinity with their familial roots. In fact, these individuals may think of themselves as a breed set apart—an alien species, even—and, indeed, they are. Like the Shooting Star, they possess a highly sensitive disposition and thrive only in very refined environments.

Shooting Star essence is a soothing remedy for these rare, precious souls, for it re-patterns the soul force and reconnects them to their true, cosmic origins. Once they have remembered their true identity, place of origin, and destiny, these weary wanderers are finally able to embrace earthly existence, as well as to offer their special gifts to the more earth-bound beings in their midst. At last, their experiences in the human realm become fuel for their own evolution, as the daily spectacle of human confusion and suffering awakens their tender hearts to love and compassion. Shooting Star remedy effectively assists in this process, while, simultaneously, granting the intergalactic traveler permission to acknowledge and delight in his or her unique, otherworldly assets.

This can be a wonderful remedy for children who have had an especially traumatic birth and are mightily resisting their earthly incarnation. Many of these souls are, in fact, star beings seeking a way to usher in the unique flights of spirit they have carried with them from other worlds. All in all, Shooting Star is a potent elixir for curing alienation on all levels.

Archetype
STAR CHILD

A profound initiation of epic proportions is beginning to reveal itself upon the earth and within human awareness. The time has come for a monumental shift in consciousness to occur. Yet another veil of illusion will soon be lifted from the eyes of the world and humanity will collectively experience multi-dimensional aspects of reality which are already in our midst but currently unseen. This planetary shift is of such magnitude that it will continue through the next two thousand years.

A new planetary archetype is being birthed as intelligent life forms from other galaxies and dimensions of reality have entered the earth realm. This is not a new phenomenon, but one that is now widely visible and acknowledged. Astrological aspects, polar shifts, and a quickening of human consciousness all point to this new understanding. It appears that many new beings, or "Star Children," are coming to earth to assist in this process. These luminous beings possess a fierce individuality, coupled with undaunting strength of will and character. They are called to earth at this time to be in service to humanity at a critical stage of human evolution. Their truest mission is to undo habitual patterns of human consciousness at the collective level, while dedicating their lives to building "A New World" in the wake of the old.

Healing

Shooting Star reminds you that you have come to this planet carrying many special qualities and gifts—along with a unique mission and destiny. Have you felt an increasing sense of alienation lately? As you contemplate the coming changes, as well as the role you may play in ushering them in, do you fear that you will open yourself to ridicule, ostracism, scapegoating, or even martyrdom? Perhaps you have always known that you possess special virtues, and have ached for a time when such qualities could be unleashed, revealing the unique star that you truly are.

In this card, a bouquet of Shooting Star flowers greets a new arrival on board a tiny Shooting Star ship. This newborn is, in fact, a fully conscious soul, choosing to enter earth in service to the cosmic forces of Love and Light. Currently, there are many Star Children on earth who have not yet remembered their true identities and reasons for being here. As more and more remember, however, they, too, will be recognized and greeted by kindred spirits. Are you remembering? Perhaps you are in the process of birthing a little being of light. It is, indeed, a privilege to be granted such an opportunity. Always remember "You can wish upon a star."

Practical Application

A large portion of humanity suffers from feelings of profound alienation. Individuals who are quite competent, even brilliant, in their professional lives will come to me complaining of an unrelenting sense of loneliness, or out-of-syncness, the origins of which are somewhat elusive. As I journey deeper with a particular client, it is often revealed that there is something highly unusual and uniquely wonderful about this person, some rare combination of qualities and interests that make for a very special gift. Along with this gift often comes much suffering, associated with feelings of invisibility at the deepest possible level, combined with a potent longing to be truly seen and affirmed. Shooting Star has proven itself an excellent remedy for the individual suffering in this way, perhaps because like the starship-shaped flower, he or she seems to have zoomed into the Earth realm for some very special, but not altogether obvious, reason. This essence offers a potent reminder and celebration of one's distant origins and unique perceptions and talents.

For example, one client, Steven, a very successful businessman by the name of Steven, came to me feeling broken and vulnerable on the inside though outwardly he appeared confident and self-assured. While accepted by his work associates, he felt completely alone in the world. He suffered from the sense that no one really knew him, that he could not reveal his True Self to others.

I prescribed Shooting Star for Steve, and suggested that he spend some time everyday writing a dialogue with himself in his journal. The proposed dialogue would be between his business persona, on the one hand, and his unique and so-called "eccentric" self, on the other. My assumption was that as he continued to take the Shooting Star essence, the more submerged aspects of himself would begin to come to the fore, and, furthermore, that this shift would be reflected in the dialogue he was having with himself. Sure enough, he reported back in three weeks, confirming that the use of Shooting Star had opened doors to his inner longing to be heard and seen, and that he carried within himself latent talents and gifts that he was afraid to acknowledge. He continued to take Shooting Star essence for three more weeks, and the next time he came in, instead of wearing his suit and tie, he had on a more casual attire and seemed at peace with himself. He had new ideas of how to make his work more interesting, but most of all, he was beginning to pursue interests that reflected his True Self. One year later, although Steve is still an accomplished businessman, he has become very active in the theater arts and is pursuing his interest in acting.

Another compelling story involves an unborn child. This is a personal testimony. During the first five months of my last pregnancy, I had increasing labor pains and pressure and was fearful that I would lose the baby. When I tested myself for essences, I found that I needed Shooting Star. As I sat in stillness, asking the Shooting Star to help me understand why I needed this particular essence, I heard a very distinct voice from the baby I was carrying. The words were "I am afraid to come to Earth. I have very special talents and gifts, and I do not think the Earth is ready for me. I want to go back home." I understood then that I needed to take the Shooting Star remedy for the unborn child, to give her the strength and courage to incarnate and fulfill her unique destiny. Within three weeks the contractions had stopped, and by my seventh month of pregnancy, I was confident that all was well. Indeed, all *was* well. Sophie was carried to term and delivered without any further complications.

After the fact, Sophie's astrology birth chart helped me understand why she was reluctant to incarnate. I have much compassion for my double Aquarius daughter, who has many planets in Aquarius, and was born during an exact Uranus/Neptune conjunction. Many children born with this configuration have highly sensitive nervous systems and have come to fulfill a very distinct mission in the new Millennium. If you know of a child born between 1992 and 1995, he or she may be in need of Shooting Star elixir.

Sagebrush

LATIN: Artemisia caucasica

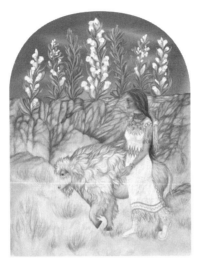

Blessing

Sagebrush, Holy Herb,
Empty my soul,
Your yellow flowers are stars in the night,
My ignorance and suffering are brought to light.

Plant Signature

*A*n evergreen shrub or woody perennial, the Sagebrush plant is distinguished by its interesting leaf patterns, silvery gray or white aromatic foliage, and small yellow flowers. This hardy plant utilizes the full strength of the sun and can tolerate extremes of heat and cold. Dried and bundled, its leaves are woven into sticks of incense which have traditionally been used by Native American tribes for the purpose of ritual cleansing.

Flower Essence

This woody perennial is one of Mother Nature's most popular healing agents for the purification of heart, mind and body—both as a flower essence and as a sacred herb. In the Native American Sweat Lodge ceremony, for example, the body of each participant is reverently "saged," or anointed with Sagebrush smoke, so that the seeker may be cleansed of all impurities in preparation for an encounter with the Great Spirit, or Wakan Tanka. Likewise, during every Native American Sundance ritual, the tribal elders wear Sage upon their heads as a sign that their minds and hearts are in close proximity to the Great Spirit's power.

The flower essence derived from Sagebrush blossoms accelerates personal evolution, for these tiny, yellow flowers act as mini suns, blooming like rays of new consciousness from its silvery green foliage and radiating the light of the Great Spirit within the heart of humanity. This potent elixir helps empty the mind, bringing the individual closer to his or her True Self, as well as to the essential teachings and wisdom of the Holy Powers. A wonderful companion on the journey of transformation, Sagebrush essence serves as a spiritual cleanser and tonic, clearing out the obstacles, illusions, and habitual patterns which typically cloud reality.

Archetype
WHITE BUFFALO CALF WOMAN

According to Lakota teachings, White Buffalo Calf Woman is associated with the mysteries of the Sacred Pipe. As legend has it, she first appeared over a distant mountain ridge, offering her beautiful, radiant, mysterious image to two awe-struck Lakota warriors. One had lustful intentions as he gazed upon her perfect form, while the other immediately recognized her as a prophetic messenger—a Wakan, or Holy Woman. As White Buffalo Calf Woman approached the warrior with impure intentions, a great cloud descended upon them, and when it lifted, all that remained of the man was his skeleton writhing with snakes. The Lakota of pure heart and mind was then summoned by this great messenger and told to announce her arrival to his tribe's chief.

Upon being introduced to the Lakota chief, White Buffalo Calf Woman removed a Sacred Pipe from the bundle on her back and offered it to him. Holding it in her two hands, the stem turned toward the heavens, she spoke, "Behold this and always love it! It is Ula Wakan (very sacred) and you must treat it as such. No impure man should ever be allowed to see it." Afterwards, she gave teachings regarding the cycles of the earth's evolution. She also introduced an awareness of the sacredness of all life: the four-leggeds; the winged birds; grandmother and grandfather earth wisdom; and all that grows upon the earth. Finally, she brought order to all the things of the universe.

As White Buffalo Calf Woman approached the ridge of a distant mountain, after leaving the company of the chief, the Lakota warrior watched her image change from that of a white buffalo calf to a black buffalo. She then disappeared behind the mountain.

Healing

There are times in our lives when we are faced with the choice either to realign ourselves to higher principles, through purification of thought, word, and deed, or to turn our backs on such a precious opportunity. The presence of this card indicates that you may be standing at such a crossroad in your own life. The choice you now make could take you to the core of self-realization or leave you relatively unchanged and stagnant. White Buffalo Calf Woman brings you courage to take the necessary steps to personal transformation, reminding you of the sweetness that shines within your heart. She sustains you with her abundant and unconditional love. Through her, the Wakan Tanka, or Great Spirit, comes to you, purging you of the impure intentions that have brought much suffering to your soul. You may wish to smudge your home, your body, your altar, or whatever space you use for meditation and prayer. As you seek to live your life in reverence for all of life, remember to give thanks to White Buffalo Calf Woman, the harbinger of cosmic justice, love and peace. Know that your life is capable of great transformation at this time.

Practical Application

In a culture that gave rise to Hollywood and high-tech, fully animated amusement parks, we are often confused about what is real and what is make believe. In healthy ways, the world of fantasy and imagination is fascinating and entertaining, and can offer us an occasional escape from the hardened edges of reality. However, the trappings of illusion can also seduce one into a life of deluded dysfunction, whether in spiritual, sexual, emotional, physical or mental realms. What we think we see is often a projection of our own longings, judgments, opinions, and expectations. Therefore, it is important to engage in a kind of ruthless truth-telling with one's self, consciously cultivating discernment and clarity, if one wishes to break the bonds of illusion. Sagebrush helps us to see through our well worn patterns, addictions, and attachments. This remedy has aided so many of my clients, for it helps eliminate negative thought forms and self-effacing habits, and purifies the aura, dispelling the fog or veil that often separates us from reality as it is.

I have recommended this essence to many people who are recognized as spiritual teachers and/or healers in the community. Danger occurs when teachers or healers become identified with the roles they have been blessed to play, and lose touch with the reality that they are but instruments through which the divine force emanates. Ego distortions cause imbalances, which in turn, create negative conditions or impaired judgment. Sagebrush has served to open the lens wider for such individuals so that they are able to see and release their attachments to personal power, prestige, fame, fortune, etc.

There are times when we seem ready to release an old habit or pattern, but are actually quite attached to the shame or guilt of it, and then get caught in the trap of self-indulgence. Remaining stuck in a pattern, going over it again and again, can retard the process of growth for which the soul is yearning. Sagebrush essence cuts through this kind of stagnation, freeing the individual to forgive and move on without self-blame or condemnation. The path to self-realization becomes broader, more realistic, more accepting of human frailties and imperfections.

Sagebrush essence, along with California Poppy, has been a wonderful combination for clients seeking to free themselves from drug addiction. Those individuals experiencing Neptune transits or with strong Neptune influences in their astrological charts can certainly benefit from the use of Sagebrush essence. It is a sacred tonic, which helps align the individual with practical dreams and grounded visions, as well as with the vertical will of his or her High Self.

Mountain Pride

LATIN: Penstemen newberryi

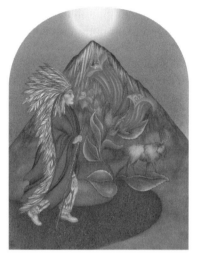

Blessing

Mountain Pride with noble beauty,
Teach me to honor my responsibility.
To walk my talk and with love impart,
To follow my journey,
A Path with Heart.

Plant Signature

*M*ountain Pride is native to the higher elevations of the Sierra Nevada Mountain range. The plant, which grows well in dry, sunny climates, has a woody base with thick, roundish, to other leaves. Its rich, rose red flowers are tubular in shape.

Flower Essence

The tubularity of Mountain Pride flowers denotes a trumpet's call to action, while their deep red color suggests a profound love of humanity, and the plant's thick base symbolizes the grounding and stabilizing of energy. The beautiful essence derived from this plant imparts an open-hearted healing response to the needs of the world, allowing the individual to face the challenges of society's imperfections in a positive, practical manner. One's motivations become pure and honest, and one is empowered to speak from the heart, as well as to act with conviction and common sense, in order to achieve his or her destiny. Any individual who commits to this path will surely promote peace in all undertakings.

Archetype
THE SPIRITUAL WARRIOR

Through the generosity of numerous Native American elders, who act as a bridge between the wisdom teachings of their ancestral traditions and the modern world, we have been blessed with many ancient Medicine stories. In this way, we are introduced to the Spiritual Warrior—also known as the Peaceful Warrior—whose primary function is spiritual in nature. Though not a warring being in the literal sense, the Peaceful Warrior is also not passive, for he is spiritually guided into various warrior-like maneuvers when no other alternative exists. Like the wrathful deities of the Tibetan Buddhist pantheon, the Spiritual Warrior of Native American legend is motivated by infinite compassion for the suffering of all beings—even the most stubborn and intractable—to help alleviate such suffering by whatever skillful means necessary. When you fail to respond to the gentle lessons life repeatedly offers you, the Spiritual Warrior presents you with more and more insistent ones until you are forced to give them the attention they deserve.

Most assuredly, the Spiritual Warrior "walks his talk" and follows through with his commitments. Taking full responsibility for his own actions, he has the authority and freedom to follow his own destiny and live the "Path of Heart." With a heart full of beauty, wisdom, and love, he receives the sacred messages of Mother Earth.

Healing

You are a Spiritual Warrior. Male or female, you carry the Medicine Way within you, for you walk in reverence as you pursue your heart's calling—your destiny. The Great Mountain and the Zenith Sun remind you of the goals you wish to accomplish. Eagle is your guide, representing the illumination of your spirit. Elk stands as your companion, noble and strong, lending its Medicine of perseverance and endurance. The Warrior wears a red cloak, the color of Mountain Pride, for he has been initiated with true, spiritual pride into the service of the world. Whatever your race, gender, age, or creed, you are being shown the paradoxical way of peaceful force. Mother Earth opens her lands for you to walk your noble journey.

Practical Application

One of the most common frustrations my clients bring to me is their confusion and lack of inspiration regarding their true callings. We have not been taught to read the inner road map of our Soul, and thus we get lost in the outer world which we have been conditioned to believe holds all the answers. The inner voice is often silenced with doubt, so it becomes my job and privilege to help guide my clients to their Higher Inner Knowing with the help of astrology and flower essences. In this regard, Mountain Pride essence can lend courage to the committed spiritual seeker. It can help one become acquainted with the warrior/warrioress within. It can teach when to be passive and when to defend, when to push for-ward and when to surrender, when to give and when to receive. These are virtues of one who listens from the heart, fully recognizing and embracing his or her destiny.

Mountain Pride has proven itself a true ally for anyone

seeking to gain a deeper union with the path he or she is here to walk. If one is pushing too hard, Mountain Pride settles the Soul, and teaches the gift of receptivity. If one is stuck, unable to move forward, Mountain Pride opens the gate to the inner path of Wisdom. Often people report a firm and solid meeting with a new way of being in the world that they had not previously considered possible.

I have given Mountain Pride to couples as a tool for improving or correcting a relationship, especially those who wish to walk a path toward a common goal together. The essence teaches good listening skills and fair play. It has been useful for individuals starting a business or venturing on a new job. It is also a great tonic for people who frequently do public speaking, especially on issues regarding law, politics, environmental conditions, and global relations.

I have a client who is a well-established politician in another state. He calls long-distance, seeking assistance from the flowers when he is about to embark upon the lecture circuit. I am very inspired by this individual, for he is a wonderful example of the way we can blend new modalities of healing with conventional work and service. He has requested Mountain Pride many times. The first time he took the essence he felt it had an impact on his inner strength and courage. His ideal is to be able to listen to others opinions and criticisms while he remains firm and well-grounded in his own knowledge and values. He seeks to offer solutions to difficult situations in a balanced and sensitive way.

If you plan to go on a hike high up toward the summit of a mountain in order to seek inspiration and new direction to life, bring some Mountain Pride along. If you happen to be in an area where this plant grows, stop along the path and enjoy this flower. It will invite you to tell your truth, to tell it from your heart with passion and conviction. Think of Martin Luther King, Jr.'s "I Have A Dream" speech. He had no fear because he had been to the mountain top and had seen the other side. Mountain Pride offers each of us this same possibility.

Apple Blossom

LATIN: Malus communis

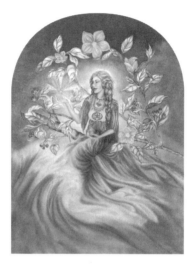

Blessing

Beautiful apple blossoms sparkle,
Like multitudes of tiny stars.
Teach me hope and faith, I pray,
So that I may offer your cosmic riches,
Each and every earthly day.

Plant Signature

The great apple tree, with its knotted wood and thick bows and branches, has an ancient and mysterious history. Found in temperate zones, it reaches perfection in cooler regions. In the spring, the apple tree produces blossoms in delicate pink and pure, five-petaled, white varieties. By their delightful fragrance and store of nectar, they attract swarms of bees. As a result of the fertilization effected by these little visitors, the tree's fruit develops, becoming in autumn the succulent, ripe apple.

Flower Essence

The apple blossom essence is a beautiful remedy which penetrates deep into one's core. Once there, it facilitates the transformative process of cycling through never-ending spirals of death and rebirth. This elixir purifies the emotions, assists the body in ridding itself of poisons from the past, and restores hope to one's inner life. In addition, it sparks a kind of star-like magic which permeates body and soul, helping to awaken trust in the innate health of the spirit. The sublime sweetness of apple blossom essence infuses the soul body with a translucent, pink light, cleansing the aura so that we may become living, holographic earth-stars—manifesting our way into abundant joy and cherishing our bodies of light.

Archetype
ASTARTE, QUEEN OF THE STARS

Astarte, The Heavenly or Holy One, was also known as Ishara, Istar, and Ashtoreth. To the Greeks, she was Aphrodite; to the Arabs, the Goddess Athtar, or "Venus in the Morning." In Aranaie, she was Ahai-Samagin, or "Morning Star of Heaven." To the Israelites, she was the Queen of Heaven to whom they offered incense, wine and cakes. Initiates traveled vast distances on pilgrimage to her great shrines in Byblos and Aphaca, both of which date back to the Neolithic period. Astarte was the "true sovereign of the world," perpetually destroying the old in order to give rise to the new. She ruled over all the stars in the heavens, and as the mother of all star-children, gave birth to the mysterious prototype of the Virgin Mary.

It is well-known today that the apple holds the hidden symbol of the star, a pentagram, in its center. For this reason, the apple, as well as the five-petaled apple blossom, are closely associated with the creative cycles of Astarte, the Star Queen, and were originally sacred to all Goddesses. Magic apples of immortality, or of death and rebirth, are common to most Indo-European mythologies. In her Garden of Paradise, Mother Hera fed the gods on apples from the Tree of Life. We find a beautiful correlation between Astarte, Mary, and Aphrodite in Romanian folklore. In this ancient context, Astarte appeared as "the Fairy Magdelana," sitting in a cosmic apple tree whose branches touched the sky and whose roots were buried in the ocean's floor.

Healing

You are offered a "star-filled" gift from the Apple Blossom. Astarte's association with Aphrodite and Venus, "the Morning Star," highlights the power of immense love and hope available to you during times of creative transformation. In Native American mythology, the Evening Star, wata-jis, heralds the emergence of the Starry Medicine Bowl in its full glory. Its presence is thought to offer a glimpse into the profound mysteries of life, death and rebirth. In many cultures, stars have come to represent hope, birth, and change. Astarte, for example, holds the golden star, while gazing with wonder into its magical depths, for she knows that the star is never stagnant. Five is the number of creative change, holding all potential within its holographic form. The star resides within the apple, a symbol of the feminine. Just as you must bite into an apple in order to expose its buried treasure, the star, you must also go to the intuitive core of your psyche in order to re-imagine and create life anew. The star of hope that Astarte offers is not the whole answer, but in some elusive way, hope ushers in faith, and deep in our hearts we begin to believe that our "Morning Star will rise again."

The apple blossoms surrounding Astarte represent the flowering potential that is yours and yours alone. The medicine of the great Bowl of Stars surrounds you, as the cosmic canopy of lighted stars manifests visions of new hope. Deep in your own heart of hearts, lives the star Queen's love, rich and plentiful, helping you to cleanse your soul aura and emerge vibrant and healthy.

Practical Application

The Apple essence I use most frequently is the Crab Apple. When the Apple tree is in full bloom, with it's tiny star-like flowers, there is no better time to make an essence. The Apple tree is one of the forces of nature most engaged with the soul of humanity. Our connection to the apple is mythical as well as mundane. Generally, it functions as a symbol of purity. The popular saying "An apple a day keeps the doctor away" was embedded in our minds as little children, and mom's homemade apple pie has become a national symbol of all that is good in America. Finally, there is the myth of Eve and that fateful bite into the apple in the Garden of Eden.

This wonderful essence acts as a purifying tonic in many ways. I have seen a blend of Manzanita and Apple Blossom work wonders as a remedy for women who feel shame about their bodies; whether the shame is related to feeling overweight or malformed in some way, or having a skin condition or an eating disorder. You can add Apple Blossom essence to your bath water, rub it on your body, drink it, and spray it around your living space from a spritzer bottle. I spray my office with Apple essence often to alleviate the stagnation in the air, and cleanse the environment.

People who are genetically sensitive, blush easily, and react strongly to stress situations sometimes develop a condition called Rosacea, referred to as adult acne by some dermatologists. This is a challenging malady, for it causes a redness of the skin and sometimes a ruddy rash that is difficult to clear. Whether you're dealing with this condition, actual acne, or a skin rash, Crab Apple essence is a very good remedy. Also, pure apple cider vinegar is reportedly effective in clearing skin rashes. Crab Apple mixed with Elm and Lavender essence can help one cope with stress and reduce skin reactions. This combination is an especially potent cleansing tonic, so if you are coming down with a cold, take some of it immediately as it will help you detox your body.

If you are just beginning to experiment with attuning to the Devic or Fairy world, try a special meeting with an apple tree. Sitting with my back against the trunk of my favorite apple tree, I often feel the rush of earthly nourishment and blessings that this shady protector has to offer.

A beautiful essence can be made by placing several blossoms from a flowering apple tree into a clear bowl of spring water. Place the bowl under the tree in a spot where the sun shines through its foliage. Imagine multitudes of stars surrounding you and showering you with abundance as you sit with this sweet bowl of flowers. In three hours time (three is the number of the Goddess), gently scoop away the flowers with a sterile instrument and add as much brandy as you have remaining water. Add several drops of this Mother Essence to apple cider in the winter for a purifying tonic. I have also made a daytime treat for my daughter, Sophie, by slicing apples and sprinkling them with Apple essence. She can then dip the fresh apple pieces in raw honey and cinnamon. She loves this treat, and it cleanses her aura and makes her cheeks rosy.

Along with its purifying qualities, Apple Blossom essence, on the etheric level, reminds us that we are pure beings of light, and that our origins are embedded in and mirrored by the twinkling stars of heaven.

California Poppy

LATIN: *Eschscholzia californica*

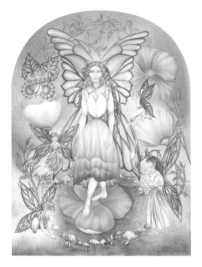

Blessing

Oh, Fairy Queen, your magical world,
Dances in my sunlit soul.
California Poppy of vibrant rays,
Teach me the fairy ways.

Plant Signature

The California Poppy is a perennial plant, native to California and Oregon, where it grows in abundance along hillsides, in country gardens and meadows, and across vast open fields. The plant grows in bright sunlight, and is quite durable in the hot summer months. Its stems, which are eight to twenty-four inches long with blue-green leaves, support soft, satiny petals, ranging in color from pale yellow to deep orange. Often referred to as a "cup of gold," the golden poppy blossom serves as a natural symbol of prosperity in the Golden State of California, where many came to find their fortunes during the Gold Rush days of the mid-1800's. Its blooms close on cloudy days and at night.

Flower Essence

The flower remedy derived from the California Poppy carries within it the radiant heights of summer and the majesty of the Sunlight. Drawing the awakened Sun force upward through the human heart, it sparks a luscious "cup of gold" within the Soul. This magic elixir also expands one's vision to include the auric antics of the fairy people, helping human beings to unite with these kindred spirits of the Devic (angelic) kingdom. For those who are naturally sensitive to such energies, this remedy helps to strengthen the connection, grounding and stabilizing the enchantment of the fairy realm at the cosmic core of one's life. Those who wish to become more sensitive to the forces of nature, are advised to take California Poppy essence in a peaceful, natural setting each day for several months. In this way, one will gradually begin to perceive the auras surrounding flowers, plants and trees, animals, human beings, and other beings found in nature.

Archetype
DEVA, THE FLOWER FAIRIES

Global myths, folklore, and fairy tales ignite the imagination and spark inquiries of a mystical nature regarding the existence of gnomes, devas, fairies, brownies, angels, elves, and the like. These magical beings of etheric beauty are the omnipresent agents of Creative Will, the engineers of Nature. As such, they direct, build, weave, and sustain all natural forces: solar, planetary, and universal. The countenance of their faces is beyond the scope of human beauty, for they possess a consciousness superseding that of

144

humanity, which emanates from them in vibrant hues and radiant auras. They are the "shining ones," or devas—self-luminous beings of iridescent light, color and energy.

Although these joyous beings are invisible to the vast majority of humans, most people can develop the refinement to sense and perceive the fairy world, but they must cultivate a purity of heart and mind, as well as genuine caring for the plants, flowers, and trees. All fairy folk have the ability to reveal themselves if they wish, and will often appear in whatever form is expected of them. Children encounter these delightful beings naturally, and are often protected by them when out in nature. Many healers, seers, artists, and poets are able to contact nature spirits due to their highly sensitive energy fields. One is most likely to attract the presence of the devas in wild flower gardens, herb gardens, meadows and glens adorned with spring flowers, forest floors moist with moss and tiny flora, and at the base of loving trees covered with many colored blossoms.

Healing

The fairy world, in its supreme purity, has come to greet you today. Perhaps you are being rewarded for having opened your heart to the wonders of the natural world. The Little People wish to pay their respects and welcome you into their magical world. Rejoice. This is, indeed, an honor. Greater vision is offered to you at this time, for you have been met with the devic consciousness of the Golden Poppy Fairy, who overlights her helpers, carrying the treasure of the warm and nurturing Sunlight within her heart. Close your eyes and allow the rapture of her radiant enchantment to fill your own loving heart. She may make herself known to you as you sleep, in meditation, or in awakened moments of ordinary life. Since fairy folk cannot resist the allure of creative energy, perhaps the Poppy Fairy will join you in your own symphony of creative harmonies as you undertake that creative project for which you've been meaning to find the time.

Practical Application

It has been interesting to observe how frequently California Poppy comes up in flower essence sessions. It has such a variety of uses that sometimes I wonder if I have made a mistake. However, when I and the client explore the flower diagnoses together, this Poppy always seems to be the perfect remedy or addition to his or her blend of flowers.

California Poppy essence is, literally, a little "cup of gold," for it holds the energetic pattern of those regions of the West where gold was discovered and fortunes made. This essence opens channels or veins within the psyche to help us explore and discover the fortunes of our inner landscape, be they psychic gifts, the ability to communicate with flowers, greater dream recall, or enhancement in writing and music talent. I have seen this essence assist clients in all of these areas.

A young woman named Lisa came into my office very tired and worn to the wick. She had just had an abortion, was attempting to heal from an eating disorder, and was trying to finish her last semester of college. California Poppy essence was strongly indicated for her. I was a bit perplexed by this, so I asked her if she was involved with drugs of some kind. She then shared that she was smoking marijuana everyday, and couldn't find the will to quit. This seemed to be the underlying issue that her subconscious needed to address. Her astral body was numb and very much out of focus.

California Poppy can be very helpful in aiding individuals move beyond addictions and glamour. I suggested Lisa take the Poppy blended with Elm and Morning Glory essence, and come back in three weeks for a re-check. When she returned, she looked like a different person. Her eyes were bright, and she reported having several dreams that opened her eyes to the new direction that she wanted her life to go. Every three weeks, for almost a year, this young woman came in for a re-check on flowers. The progress she made was remarkable, and, she is now apprenticing with me as a flower essence practitioner so that she can administer flower essences to her own clients. She is also studying to become a psychologist. She feels California Poppy essence made it possible for her to access her inner world of dreams and visions, and to wake up to her special calling in life.

Groups of people sometimes gather to explore the possibilities of telepathy and astral travel. Periodically, someone will ask me if I can suggest particular flower essences to facilitate this type of exploration. I often recommend California Poppy as one such flower helper. I have used it myself when seeking attunement with a particular writing project or creative endeavor. In fact, I took California Poppy quite often while creating the Power of Flower Cards, and feel certain that on several occasions this essence helped me make contact with what I like to call the Fairy Queen of Nature. The Fairy Queen is so willing to share her secrets of nature with me, sending shimmering rays of glowing color through my body, in the process. For this reason, I connected the California Poppy with the Fairy Queen. She is one of my closest allies.

Orchid

LATIN: Bauhinia forticata

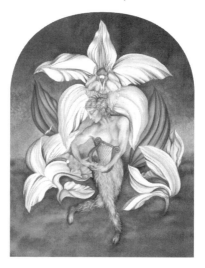

Blessing

In the ecstasy of Nature,
Through the soul of Pan,
May the Orchid refine,
The earthly human,
Orchid's pure essence
Awakens the heart.
Sexuality and Love
Are never apart.

Plant Signature

The orchid tree is a dark green evergreen, native to Brazil. Regarded as the hardiest of the Bauhinia, it has been known to reach a height of twenty feet. With twisting trunk and prickly thorns, nestled in sharply-angled branch joints, this tree is striking in appearance. Through the spring and summer months, it bears narrow-petaled, creamy white flowers which grow up to three inches wide. Its blossoms reach for the light yet are very sensitive to direct sun, doing best in semi-shady areas.

Flower Essence

An extremely potent flower elixir, Orchid is known to greatly enhance one's attunement to nature's enraptured sensuality and divine procreative forces. In fact, Pliny, an early botanist, claimed that even holding the roots in one's hands would arouse one to sexual ecstasy. It is not surprising, then, that parts of the orchid plant were common ingredients in love potions, nor that in the language of flowers, a man gave a woman an orchid as a sign of seduction. Orchid essence, however, seeks to refine the raw drive of sexual desire, for its white flowers symbolize purity, while its thorns represent the pain that accompanies the desecration of sexuality. Orchid and Rose elixirs—both from thorny plants associated with love—make a beautiful blend which is highly recommended for couples seeking spiritual/sexual union.

Archetype
PAN, GOD OF WILD NATURE

The word orchid comes from the Greek, *orchis*, meaning testicle, because of its twin bulbs resembling testicles. The Romans named the orchid "satyrion," claiming it grew from semen left on the ground by the Satyrs—fawn like beings considered an embodiment of the horned god of wild nature, known to the Greeks as Pan. Since Pan was identified with unbridled sexuality and desire, he was regarded as evil by the Christian authorities of ancient times. Hence, his cult was suppressed.

With twisting ram horns atop his head—much like the twisted trunk of the orchid tree—the Roman Satyr resembled the Egyptian god Amn-Ra, whom the Greeks considered another aspect of Pan. Closely associated with the Cult of Dionysus, Pan is said to have mated with the great Goddesses Athena, Penelope, and Selene.

By the 19th century, Pan's image was somewhat sanitized by the refining lenses of poets, naturalists, and romantics who saw him as a gentle being embodying the wild aspects of nature and humanity. In their artistic depictions, Pan roamed the woods unsullied by the corrupting influence of civilization—free of the kind of degradation wrought by the Industrial Revolution. In the modern day mythology of the U.S. men's movement, especially as expressed during ritual retreats in wooded settings, Pan is revered as the male patron of nature.

However, archeological evidence suggests that Pan may have actually begun his legendary life as the Hindu fertility God Pancika, consort to one of the primal Mother Goddesses Hariti, who suckled hundreds of pre-Vedic animal spirits. Just as men can only reach full maturity through healing relationships with women—relationships which heal the primal disconnection with their mothers—it may be that Pan, the ultimate confirmed bachelor, will only reach his maturity as a cultural icon when he is understood first and foremost in his role as a consort to the Goddess. Only then can his ritual re-enactment truly open the gate to Mother Nature's sensual garden, for men and women alike.

Healing

The forces of nature are vibrantly alive with ultraviolet colors and wave frequencies which we as humans cannot perceive. The same is true with regards to your own inner gardens of sexuality. With the appearance of Pan, the Wild God of the forest, you are offered a mythical perspective on your own primal nature and instincts, ushering in a higher awareness regarding these matters.

The orchid tree fine tunes itself, redefining its form over and over again amongst its own thorns and convoluted pathways. Its luscious flowers can twist, bend, lean, and climb when seeking the light, but they remain succulent in the shade. Their blooms will shrivel up and die if exposed for too long to the heat of direct sunlight. Your sexuality is like that, too. You must, with constant striving, seek the highest, fullest expression of your passions, and, yet, learn to temper them, as well. And, like the orchid tree, you too, must find your way amongst thorns and tortured pathways until you come to rest in the pure realization of your Divine Sexual Nature, symbolized here by the Orchid flower.

Practical Application

I often use Orchid essence with couples when they are seeking deeper union with each other. Using the chakras of the body as access points, I have the couple apply this essence on the different chakras at periodic intervals in order to trigger receptivity and oneness. For the male, Orchid essence seems especially beneficial on the heart chakra; for the female, on the throat chakra. Both should apply the essence on the creative second chakra, and solar plexus, third chakra. The gift of the essence is subtle. It transmutes what would normally be registered as primal sexual energy into subtle vibrations of pure bliss and ecstasy. Applying this essence on intimate sexual areas is very beautiful, as well.

A blend of Orchid, California Poppy, and Angelica was used at a flower essence workshop which I facilitated. The entire group took the essence together, and our attunement was a pure delight to behold. Each person was instructed to go out into Nature and choose a flower, tree, or plant to connect and commune with. The California Poppy essence invoked the ability to hear the beautiful stories of the flowers, the Orchid essence brought one's attention to the element of Pan, and the Angelica essence grounded the experience into human understanding. The Orchid essence is one I like to offer to students who are just beginning to listen to Nature.

Fig

LATIN: Ficus carica

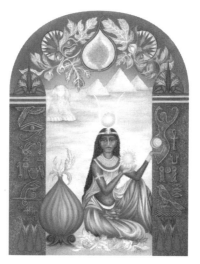

Blessing

Sacred fig,
You carry seeds of feminine delight,
Fiery flowers of masculine light.
Alchemical vessel within my soul,
Reveal your secrets—make me whole.

Plant Signature

The fig was originally known to exist in ancient Egypt, where it was prominent in the mythology of the region, and is said to have been transported to Europe by the Romans. The fig tree typically lives to a ripe old age, producing an abundant supply of figs—which are nestled in the axils of its wide and bushy leaves—over the course of its long life. Neither fruit nor flower, the fig is a remarkable plant. What is commonly referred to as the "fruit" of the fig is, in fact, its syncarp (a fleshy receptacle, inside of which are scores of tiny male and female flowers). Miraculously, these flowers mature and blossom wholly in the fig's dark interior. Its female flowers eventually develop into "seeds," and it is these seeds which are actually the fruit of the plant. Pollination is accomplished by wasps so tiny that they are able to crawl into the plant's receptacle. Not surprisingly, the fig stands alone in this peculiar arrangement.

Flower Essence

When laid open, the fig has been said to resemble the human brain, providing an important clue as to the healing properties of its essence. Made using the fruit flower and seed of the fig, this profound elixir is capable of restoring and enhancing memory, and thus is an excellent remedy when doing past-life or early-childhood regression work. Fig essence also balances one's male and female elements at the cellular level; bringing the right and left hemispheres of the brain into a state of equilibrium, while helping the individual to achieve greater clarity, and, ultimately, gain access to higher aspects of Mind. In addition, it restores deep wisdom to the body, and, in particular, can raise one's awareness regarding conception. The fig elixir is a rare juice. Use it sparingly and with great reverence, giving thanks to the Goddess for this unusual gift of nature.

Archetype
ISIS

According to Egyptian scripture, "In the beginning there was Isis, Oldest of the Old. She was the Goddess from whom all becoming arose." Within the temple of her sacred womb, she held the many precious secrets of alchemical magic. Out of this mysterious vessel, she birthed the sun and moon, as well as all aspects of life: heaven and earth;

male and female. In Egyptian mythology, Isis was given occult knowledge by a great angel and instructed to keep it to herself. She told only her son Horus, who was the living light—her begotten son—birthed from her all-knowing Self. Hermetic texts, with their basis in Egyptian mythology, depict Isis as having revealed the mysteries of the stars to God, Himself. Her deep insights gave rise to the phrase "As above, so below," for Isis plants star knowledge into the heart of humanity. Revered as Nature, Herself, she is the living embodiment of divine wisdom, for she is never apart from its infinite variations in the natural world. Her existence is a sacrament, furthering the cause of human evolution.

Isis' temple walls are etched with hieroglyphic portrayals of the ancient language of space and time. The many holographic patterns and geometric shapes depicted there echo through our bodies into eternity. Symbols of the heart, eternity, life, truth, justice, and soul are inscribed on her garden gates, along with the spirit image of the sacred feminine. On her right arm she wears the ankh, a universal life charm, and in her hands she holds the unifying polarities—the sacred sun and the holy moon. Her vessel sprouts with life, as new forms of love and wisdom gestate and flower.

Healing

The fig is a rare plant, containing tiny seeds and flowers within a receptacle, just as Isis is a rare Goddess associated with a sacred vessel containing alchemical secrets. When Isis makes her appearance to you today, she opens the channels of your Higher Mind, decoding the memory of your deepest origins which can tell you her many secrets. The luscious fig overhead is opened, revealing the inner fruits and nectars that are stored within your soul.

The Holy Tree of Life at Mataria in Egypt, sacred to Isis, was the wild fig tree. Dried figs and wood from its holy branches were placed in the tombs of early dynasties to serve as womb symbols for rebirth. According to Ananda Tantra, the fig leaf is a form of the yoni. No doubt, the fig and Isis appear to you as enlightened messages of the divine feminine. Her vessel of life pours forth the elixir of all potentials; like Isis, you are granted the secrets of alchemy. Be still...Her flowers blossom in the vessel of your own heart.

Practical Application

Fig essence is one of my favorites, for, like the Apple, the mythology surrounding the Fig has roots that extend into the inner recesses of human anatomy. When I first decided to make a Fig essence many years ago, I was intrigued to realize that the Fig tree did not produce flowers like other fruit trees, but, instead, created little womb-like containers, the Fig, and within this matrix, the flower would bloom. Since the Fig is a tiny womb, itself, it is easy to see how Fig essence might be useful in furthering the cause of human procreation.

In fact, I have used Fig essence over and over again for those seeking to conceive a child, as it acts as an agent or messenger from the High Self to the reproductive organs. If a man and a woman are seeking conception using the natural method of intercourse, then I have them take the essence together. If the couple is two women, or, if this is a single woman seeking conception through artificial insemination, I like to use essences that will wrap the women in an energy field of nurturance and love. When tracking the ovulation cycle, I have them take Fig essence the day before they plan to conceive. In addition, I usually have them take Pomegranate essence the week before, mixed with a specific remedy that matches the personal needs of the individual. Flowers that address fear, resistance, and any other unconscious malady that may be blocking conception are often indicated.

The womb-like Fig also bears a resemblance to the human brain, and thus, as a plant medicine, it helps one to access visions and manifestations. Likewise, it helps with the conception process for those who are finding it difficult to conceive due to some sort of unconscious blockage in the mental body. The air, or intellectual qualities, have stifled the flow of watery receptivity. Unfortunately, some people feel shame and guilt concerning their difficulty in conceiving, and so I administer essences to help with this, as well. Otherwise, another obstacle will block the flow. Flowers alone cannot determine whether or not a woman will conceive. A greater will and the force of her Higher Self will also play a role in the process. Again, flowers are mere helpers in a grander scheme of life tapestry.

Black Cohosh

LATIN: Cimicifuga racemosa

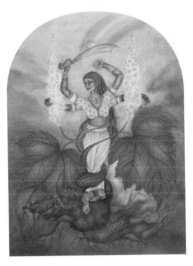

Blessing

Black Cohosh with gnarly roots,
Offering flowers of tender white shoots,
Kali Ma reveals her sword,
Breaking the ties, cutting the cords.
All my demons are eternally free—
Black Cohosh, you transform me.

Plant Signature

*A*lso known as Black Snake Root, Rattle Root, and Squaw Root, Black Cohosh is a summer plant found in shady woods, as well as on their periphery. "Cohosh" is an Indian word for "rough" and "black," referring to the plant's gnarled and knotty roots which extend deep into the ground. In contrast, its pointed white flowers spike upward toward the light.

Flower Essence

This plant has powerful healing properties symbolized by its pure, white flowers which embody the power of transformation as they blossom out of dark and tangled roots under the crust of the earth. Referred to as a "woman's plant" for its estrogen-like qualities, which soothe menstrual cramps and assist in child birth, Black Cohosh is as effective as an herb tincture as it is a flower essence. In its herbal form, it must be used with great caution.

As a flower essence, Black Cohosh envelopes and balances the emotional and mental realms, guiding the individual through desired transformations. This elixir also helps one find the necessary inner resources—such as courage and strength—for overcoming addictive patterns and emotional dependencies which can undermine self-confidence and self-esteem. With its gentle assistance, the dark, deeply-buried, gnarly roots of past traumas are more easily untangled, unleashing repressed tendencies, and in the process, igniting an enormous healing journey of energetic transmutation. True liberation can follow, as the soul gives rise to a luminous bouquet of purity which is one's essential, divine self, reborn.

Archetype
KALI, THE GODDESS OF DESTRUCTION

Kali is also known as Shakti, or Kali Ma. She is the embodiment of pure female energy for she is the deepest void or womb, where all is born, must die, and be born again. Most commonly depicted as a black, warrior Goddess with striking features, Kali is a fierce protector of the universe. Her task is to strip away, cut back, and devour all obstructions and hindrances—hence, she is typically associated with the fearful imagery of transmutation, such as a sword held in one of her four arms, and snakes and skulls dangling from her body. In seeming contrast, two of her arms reach out to bless and acknowledge her many fervent devotees, as well as to renew the seed of possible enlightenment for humanity. As the mistress of time and space, she governs the mortal dimensions of human and planetary evolution.

Healing

With this card, Kali Ma has come to serve you in the deepest possible manner. The Black Cohosh elixir is her tonic; for like her, it is born out of the dark places, revealing all that must be relinquished back to its unfathomable shadows. These healing forces come to your aid at a time of tremendous transformation. Addictive patterns, dysfunctional relationships, self-imposed suffering, and destructive habits of various kinds—all such afflictions are transformed by Black Cohosh.

Kali stands victorious amidst the rooted entanglements of despair. White flowers blossom around her, symbolizing the peace and tranquillity that inevitably arise after her raging storm. A rainbow encircles Kali's sword, while her arms offer a kind blessing. Remember, out of your deepest, darkest fears, a new cycle of evolution beckons. Your path to enlightenment is secure; Mother Kali protects you along the way.

Practical Application

Black Cohosh is a powerful herb for women. Among other things, it facilitates the balancing of hormones in pregnant and menopausal women. In the course of these two deeply transformative processes, Black Cohosh also helps a woman surrender to the necessary rhythms of birth and death. For this reason, I have always had a healthy respect for Black Cohosh, knowing that it must be used with great care and professionalism.

So, when I heard about the Black Cohosh essence, I was interested, but cautious. Also, I had such a picture of the plant as a gnarly root that I never really thought of it having a flower. I was surprised to discover that the blossom of the plant was white and sweet, extending rods of purifying transformation toward the heavens. A flower essence made of these beautiful flowers must be extremely potent, I thought, in facilitating the cutting of the twisted knots of addiction, fear, denial, and abuse. In fact, the first time I held a bottle of Black Cohosh essence in my hand, an immediate image of Kali-Ma sprung to mind. I knew this essence would be a powerful addition to my collection of elixirs.

There is no question when Black Cohosh essence is right for a person, or for that matter, when it is wrong. One should never give this essence to a person who is not ready to seriously engage with the cutting of cords, the shattering of illusions, the liberation from one's knotted, gnarly past. It is for those people who have done their work, and who are passionately committed to freedom from their own patterns and projections. This is a person who is no longer blaming, shaming, or feeling like a victim, but who is ready for the beautiful ride home to the Source, one's True Self.

A woman named Karen came to see me at a critical juncture in her life. She was a strong and intelligent woman in her mid-thirties, with a beautiful baby girl, and an abusive relationship with her husband (a man she professed to love, yet fear). She was trying to gain the courage to leave him, to start a new life, and to forgive herself for having engaged with him and his addictions. As we sat in my office, I could see that she was still attached to him; not in her mind, but in her psychic body and through her memories. With Karen's permission, we decided to do a cutting of the cord meditation, where we visualized her husband's image in a big ball above her. Slowly, at a pace with which Karen was comfortable, I led her through the process of seeing the ball moving farther and farther into the void of empty space, toward the point where she would eventually cut the cord attaching her to her husband.

When it was time to cut the cord, Karen began to panic and did not want to detach. Subsequently, she and I spent several sessions looking at her patterns of attachment and fear. Up to this point, I had not suggested Black Cohosh but had, instead, given her varying doses of Buttercup and Larch essence, plus one bottle of Walnut and Pine. These helped quite a lot, but ultimately did not unravel the knot of her addiction to her husband.

Finally, one day Karen came to see me and she looked ready. I told her about Black Cohosh; that it is potent and effective, but only in combination with the deepest resolve and intent to set herself free from her past. She took Black Cohosh for only two weeks, and I was amazed at the progress she made in that amount of time. Never looking back, Karen changed her life dramatically for the better by leaving her abusive relationship. She has become a shining example of the fierce compassion of Kali-Ma, sword intact, in the real world.

Angelica

LATIN: Angelica archangelica

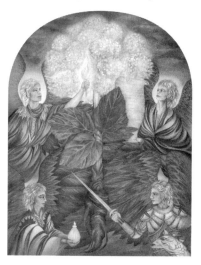

Blessing

Angelic blossom of light and mirth,
Anchor my soul,
Into the roots of the earth.
Your luminous glory,
Your halo of gold,
Help me to deepen,
This destiny I hold.

Plant Signature

*A*s its exalted name suggests, Angelica—also known as Angel Root or Archangel Root—has for centuries been held in the highest esteem by Eastern and Western healers alike for its profoundly transformative, spiritual properties.

Its root system, its primary element is anchored deep in the earth, and supports a stem of substantial proportions. It can grow up to six and a half feet in height with a circumference as thick as a human arm. The majesty of the plant is revealed in an umbrella of greenish white flowers which delicately overlight its powerful foundation.

Flower Essence

The many wonderful qualities of the Angelica plant offer humanity a lens through which to understand both the meaning of human incarnation and the truth about human potential. Its deep root system symbolizes the importance of thoroughly grounding ourselves in the earth plane, while its majestic floral umbrella represents the delicate halo of heavenly guidance and angelic protection which is always available to us. The essence derived from this most heavenly and rooted of plants, helps one establish a firm connection between the refined, subtle realm of angelic light surrounding us, and the tangible, material world which grounds and anchors us to earth. Once such a link is made, we are given the inner strength and stamina required for pursuing our life's destiny.

Archetype

THE ARCHANGELS MICHAEL, GABRIEL, URIEL, AND RAPHAEL

The Archangels Michael, Gabriel, Uriel, and Raphael—each of his own free will and each in his own unique way—offer themselves in unconditional service to humanity. These leaders of the angelic realm, have dedicated themselves to the ultimate good of the whole, making whatever sacrifices are necessary in the interest of sanctifying human existence. Surrounded by beautiful auras of heavenly light, the Archangels assist in the anchoring of humanity's soul-body to the earth plane, so that we may learn the path of service, dedication and sacrifice. In this way, they patiently lead us, step by step, upward on the path of higher consciousness.

Michael, in Hebrew, literally means "Who is God." Known as the "Captain of Heavenly Hosts" and the "Leader of the Archangels," Michael is also sometimes referred to as "The Lord of the Way." As the slayer of dragons, he helps dispel evil intentions and is the guardian of holy places. His ultimate mission is to purify.

Hebrew for "Fire of God," Uriel is the angel of prophecy who inspires ideas and visions amongst the teachers of the world. Often shown with a scroll, Uriel transforms ordinary, uninspired thoughts into reflections of the divine, and is associated with the arts and all musical endeavors.

Gabriel, whose name means "Strength of God" in Hebrew, is said to be the bearer of good news. Love is his great force, and he is often depicted carrying a lily, symbolizing purity, as well as a torch, representing the sun or solar power. Gabriel offers this light of God to all who seek rebirth. He is also shown with a trumpet, heralding the call to resurrection.

Hebrew for "God Heals" or "Divine Healer," Raphael is caretaker of the Earth's natural world, as well as of the flowering consciousness of humanity. Known as the angel of healing and mercy, he infuses all healing institutions with radiant light. Raphael carries a golden vial of soothing balm and an arrow or spear. His aim, represented by the arrow, is to heal the world.

Healing

The Archangels offer light. Even in darkness, or when attachments and distractions seduce humanity away from its Divine essence, the Archangels continually pour their protective and loving radiance into you. In this way, they strengthen your spirit so that you may persist in your goal of ascension, trusting that each earthly step brings you closer to the luminous world of the Soul. Remember this: you would not have been given an earthly body if you were not meant to anchor that which is perfect, infinite, and eternal in material form. Each incarnation in the human realm is a privilege.

Without a doubt, as you read these words you are especially close to the angelic world. Which angel is near you now? Perhaps you can identify with the qualities of a particular Archangel and invite his presence into your life at this time. The Archangels offer you a shimmering umbrella, grounding the forces of light in your human experience. Accept the gift, and by so doing, begin the journey that will surely culminate in the fulfillment of your destiny.

Practical Application

Like the Rose, the Angelica plant roots very deep, anchoring its special qualities into the earth. It activates healing on all levels, strengthens one's relationship with his or her Guardian Angel, and balances the temporal and spiritual worlds.

A woman brought her little daughter, Jennifer, in because she was ungrounded and fearful at night. We talked about what might be bothering the child. She was a very sensitive soul who seemed to have a vivid imagination. As we talked, I began to suspect that Jennifer was having more than her share of invisible, nocturnal visitors, but was reluctant to speak about this. I understood that she was being bothered by these real or imagined presences, and that she needed some extra protection during both the day and night. I gave her a dose bottle of Angelica, Lavender, and Yarrow essences. Her nerves were calmed down by the next day. She became more grounded due to the Angelica essence, while the Yarrow protected her, and the calming Lavender soothed her nerves. Jennifer's mother continued giving her Angelica essence for some time. Mother and daughter used it as a nightly ritual, invoking Jennifer's Guardian Angel, and saying a prayer for peace.

I also use Angelica essence for rituals and special blessings involving babies. I like to give a gift of Angelica to a family at the birth of a new member. When taken by the immediate family members, particularly the parents, the essence helps them commune with the baby's Angel Spirit and anchor the baby to the earth.

Angelica essence is often called for when an artist comes to me seeking inspiration from the sphere of light which surrounds him or her. Incidentally, it would seem that Renaissance painters and sculptors were embodying the essence of Angelica when they produced the glorious works of that era. I took Angelica essence with me on a trip to Italy because I knew I would be visiting many churches and museums. The six Catholic services I attended, especially the singing and the chanting, put me in another world. The statues came to life, and the movement of the images depicted in the art stirred me to tears.

I also took Angelica on the day I decided to climb up to a special grave site with a view of the Alps and a lake. Those resting in this glorious place are truly sleeping with the angels. Angelica is another essence to offer those who are crossing the threshold into death. A combination of Angel's Trumpet, Angelica, and Purple Water Lily essence will guide one safely to the other side.

Queen of the Night

LATIN: Cereus greggii

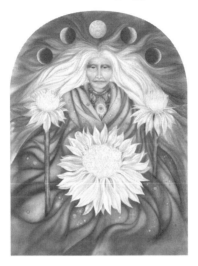

Blessing

Queen of Night,
Lunar light,
Bathe my soul tonight.
In virtue, truth, and serenity,
Let my heart be one with thee.

Plant Signature

*A*ptly named, the Queen of the Night Cactus is a luminous desert flower, that shines with a crown-like radiance in the dark of the night, closing its bloom upon sunrise. It is attached beneath the ground to an enormous root tuber that can weigh as much as eighty-five pounds. However, above ground only a skinny stem, resembling a stick, can be seen supporting its huge, fragrant white blossom.

Flower Essence

Deep within each of us lives a great store of repressed and sublimated feminine energy and wisdom, much like the subterranean tuber that supports the Queen of the Night. The elixir made from this regal desert flower assists in the balancing of one's yin qualities by opening channels to the womanly gifts and secrets which have long been buried within the soul. Just as the Queen of the Night flower shimmers in the moonlight, individuals taking her essence experience an illumination of the deep and darkened places of their psyches. For this reason, I highly recommend taking this essence at night, under the Moon, while asking for guidance from your dreams.

The Queen of the Night plant has the ability to regenerate broken stems and restore its life force. This quality of rejuvenation is imprinted in its essence, as well, making the elixir a valuable tool for women during the changing cycles of life, and offering men the courage to journey into the intuitive realm where cycles of birth, death, and rebirth prevail. Queen of the Night also helps us to age gracefully as well as to honor the subtle grace of the aged.

Archetype

GRANDMOTHER WISDOM

Historically, the wise teachings of the elders were revered by tribal members, for the stories of ancestral mystery were patterned in their souls. The Grandmothers shared the knowledge of the changing cycles and seasons, and offered the song of life to those who longed to hear the Truth. As midwives to body and soul, the Wise Women birthed the generations, issuing forth the seeds of the future. They understood that the knowledge of the Earth and her people is encoded in the plant, mineral, and animal realms, and that these realms must be honored and restored.

Through the teachings of Grandmother Wisdom, we come to know the Moon and all Her cycles. She leads the way through the Moon lit paths of our inner worlds, gently tugging at the veil of darkness. Guiding those who wish to follow her into the memory of time and space, she assists in the important work of lineage retrieval. Finally, she teaches us that every heart is filled with dreams, prayers, hopes, and faith, and that a graceful life is given to those who are grateful.

Healing

The Queen of the Night comes to you today, showering you with moonbeams of heavenly wisdom. You are crowned with the her brilliant aura as she protects and overlights your journey into the great mystery. Shining in your heart like an evening lantern, she lights your way to greater Self-Knowledge. You may wish to meditate at night, under the Moon, letting its luminous rays caress you with their soft lunar light. Teaching patience, love, and endurance, the Queen of the Night reminds you that you too, are a keeper of wisdom. Perhaps you need to be reminded of your own innate healing abilities. Perhaps it is time to focus your healing light upon yourself, in order to revitalize the storage house of your own precious energy.

Practical Application

There is something mysterious about flowers that bloom in the night. I feel these are feminine flowers, for they reach for the light of the Moon, the illumined orb that guides women through the changing cycles of our bodies and emotions. The forces of these flowers stimulate the unconscious and beckon us to find light in the darker regions of the Soul.

Queen of the Night Cactus is a very useful flower during menopause when a woman is led to explore the deep, dark well of wisdom within. Her body becomes a regenerating matrix wherein the inner seeds of creation and self renewal germinate over and over again. The focus of her life turns inward, remapping the journey of Soul fulfillment. Queen of the Night Cactus comes to many women during this cycle, as it mirrors the blossoming that happens in the mystery of the night cycle when our listening and attunement to the world is most acute.

A colleague and therapist in my city was facilitating a woman's group focused on the menopausal years. She used Queen of the Night Cactus essence with the women as they traveled through the Moon cycles together. Each woman was to track her emotions, longings, needs, inspirations, creative movement, and sexuality through the three month cycle. With the assistance of this flower elixir, the women stayed in touch with each crescent, quarter, new moon, full moon cycle and were able to track and stabilize key emotions and thought processes that occurred predictably throughout the three month cycle. They were so pleased with the results of this experiment that, on their own, many have continued to use the essence to help track their cycles. I keep a stock of Queen of the Night Cactus essence on hand for them, and take a little sip of it regularly, myself.

A young woman client named Emily, who was wise beyond her years, found it difficult to own her wisdom, fearing it would be invalidated in the world. Seeing the ancient love of grandmother wisdom in her eyes, I wanted nothing more than to validate this young woman's gift. Queen of the Night essence was the chosen remedy for Emily, along with Sunflower. The cactus essence led her to the acknowledgment of her wise self, and the Sunflower helped to balance her own identity and authority. She called me two weeks later in tears, for she had a dream visit from her beloved grandmother who had passed away some time before. Emily's grandmother looked just as the young woman remembered her, except that she now had Emily's face. As this story illustrates, Queen of the Night Cactus opens the dream cycles as well.

Saguaro Cactus

LATIN: Cereus giganteus

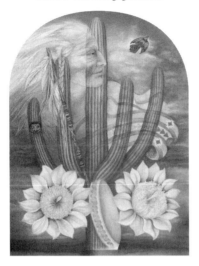

Blessing

Ancient knowledge of mystery,
Saguaro's message, living
Within this desert tree.
Strong and proud; loving and true,
My life receives protection from you.

Plant Signature

*A*n integral part of any desert scene, the Saguaro Cactus is a mighty plant, with an aura of tremendous stature and authority, known to reach the majestic height of twenty feet or more. Given its slow growing nature—approximately one foot for every fifteen years of life—a life span of 300 years is not unusual for this Grandfather of the plant world! At eight feet tall, or approximately 120 years of age, this great cactus will begin to produce flowers. The mature plant has a root system capable of holding up to 200 gallons of water—enough to sustain it for an entire year.

Flower Essence

Not surprisingly, given its great stature and majesty, this elixir can help individuals align vertically to a higher order of personal authority and integrity. Father issues, on both personal and cultural levels, are eased as one attunes to the wisdom of the inner Wise Grandfather who protects and guides his people. At the personal level, Saguaro Cactus essence is especially healing for those who have lost a father at an early age, or experienced paternal abandonment at or before birth. In the broader cultural context, this elixir acts as a powerful healing agent for the global phenomenon known as "father hunger" and balancing masculine energy in all individuals and teaching honorable ways to access and execute the Will. It is an excellent remedy to use when working with adolescent boys, and can be very beneficial for young men, in general, as it gently aligns one with the honor code of right living. Since the Saguaro Cactus takes many years to mature, this essence also teaches patience and virtue. Its use is, therefore, highly recommended for ceremony and ritual, especially where tradition and age are being honored.

Archetype
GRANDFATHER WISDOM, TIME KEEPER

Time Keepers understand that all of life is made up of certain archetypal patterns of the sort found in crystals, plants, DNA structures, earth and star formations, light frequencies, and sound. The elders, who carry time within them, understand that such patterns are imprinted in our dreams, intentions, and Self Knowing, and that they change with the growth and evolution of Earth and all the galaxies. Grandfather Wisdom patiently watches over the many offspring issuing forth from Grandmother's Sacred Womb. Buried deep in the folds of his great medicine blanket, we find the ancestral origins of all those who walk this

Earth. Likewise, in the soothing rhythm of his drum, we hear the heartbeat of the people—the pulse of life, itself, effecting all states of being. His walking staff a symbol of direction and stature, he shows us the way into our own liberating authority, while teaching us important lessons about patience and intention. Magic and power have long been associated with this staff, or walking stick. Symbolizing the Tree of Life, it serves as an axis between Heaven and Earth—a tool for taking messages skyward.

Healing

The Saguaro Cactus is a powerful healing presence. Its stature and dignity symbolize the shift you are undergoing in relation to your own personal power. The masculine principle within your psyche is rebalancing at this time, and you find yourself able to receive Grandfather Wisdom's sacred knowledge, which resides within your heart, just as it lives at the center of this proud, majestic plant. The folds of Grandfather's garment reach out to protect your Earth Walk; his drum and walking stick are visible to the external world for they are essential gifts he brings to the journey. Drumming puts us in sync with the rhythms of the cosmos, while the walking stick is a symbol of stamina and purpose. You may wish to join a drumming circle at this time, or journey through the mountains and valleys of your homeland, exploring the very nature of your own authority and will power. A tremendous amount of life force is available to you now, for, like the Saguaro Cactus, you are able to sustain your power over long periods of time. Time is your ally. Be patient and let the wisdom of your ancestral lineage guide you onward.

Practical Application

We live during a period in history when everything is sped up. Even children comment on this. As a child, I remember thinking it was forever and a lifetime before the holiday season returned. But, little ones today are faced with a fast-paced culture with almost no appreciation or understanding of natural rhythms and cycles. Grandfather Time, living within the Saguaro Cactus, comes to us in times of crisis in order to steady our lives and remind us to slow down and connect to what is truly important in life. Saguaro essence connects us to our ancestors, the land dwellers, people who watched the Sun rise and the Moon set according to the rhythms of the seasons. It is useful for people who feel ungrounded and overwhelmed by the accelerated pace of personal growth and change.

I recently had a client who needed a long-distance crisis counsel. Wendy is a very sensitive woman with great inner conviction and spiritual intention. She felt ungrounded due to the fact that changes were happening so quickly in her life. She also sensed a very significant shift occurring within her. At the end of our session, I suggested that I choose a random Power of Flower card in order to give us more information regarding her healing journey. Not surprisingly, the card that appeared was Saguaro Cactus. When I relayed this information to Wendy, she was very touched, for everyday as she took her daughter to school, she drove past a grove of Saguaro Cactus and had the sense that they were reaching out to calm and protect her. The choice of this card was all the encouragement Wendy needed. She began sitting amongst the cactus plants in order to better receive their transmission of peace and stability. I sent her a bottle of the flower essence, as well, so that she could partake of the plant's energy on every level.

Saguaro Cactus essence is also highly recommended for men who long to reconnect with a father figure or male mentor. For this reason, it is a useful essence for men's groups. I have a male client who uses Saguaro Cactus essence when he drums in his men's circles. He feels it helps him connect with the elders, and that they show him the way to the heart beat of the Earth. This essence is especially useful during Saturn transits when what is called for is a serious exploration of issues of authority and self-discipline, along with a major restructuring of one's life. Saguaro Cactus mixed with Sunflower has been given to many Saturn-challenged clients with great result.

Calla Lily

LATIN: *Zantedeschia*

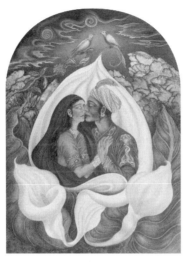

Blessing

Calla Lily, pure and white,
Yellow sun rising within her bright.
I join the cosmic, alchemical trance,
Where love becomes a tantric dance.

Plant Signature

*P*lants belonging to the Lily family are generally understood to mirror the unity between spiritual and
material realms, and are also associated with feminine and
masculine principles, respectively. The Calla Lily, for example, embodies the power and mystery of the feminine in its
large, moist bulbs, representing the world of deep feelings.
Likewise, it blossoms into a white floral vessel, symbolizing
the "cup of life." At the center of this vessel, however, stands

an erect, yellow stamen—a decidedly phallic, masculine image held within a womb-like space. The leaves of the Calla Lily twist, curl and cluster around the flower, further underscoring the quality of intimacy and integration which this Lily can bring to the soul.

Flower Essence

Unfortunately, our modern world has perpetuated a false dichotomy between the spiritual and sexual spheres, creating an atmosphere of extreme polarization. Calla Lily essence is a sublime tincture for all who wish to bridge this ancient chasm. It purifies, rejuvenates, and balances one's spiritual-sexual nature, gently reuniting masculine and feminine principles within the individual, and, thereby, expanding one's notion of sexual identity so that true androgyny can blossom within the human soul. This alchemical marriage is accomplished when sexual energy is rightly located within its all-encompassing spiritual matrix. In this way, the deep mysteries of sexuality, intimacy, and union are spiritualized. Calla Lily elixir also awakens lovers to a New World order concerning relationships—one in which it becomes imperative that we offer our complete Selves to our beloved. For many, anything less is no longer considered acceptable. Finally, this essence opens the channels for individuals and couples to fully embrace the beloved within.

Archetype
INDIAN TANTRIC LOVERS

The classical Indian treatise on the Art of Love, known as the Kama Sutra, taught its initiates the Path of Creative Energy or Tantra, whereby ecstasy, spirituality, and sexuality were harmonized and balanced. In this context, sexuality was understood as the raw material for samadhi (enlightened consciousness) because of its potential to awaken one's longing for the sweet taste of spiritual ecstasy, and was, therefore, given a place of high honor in tantric temples. The quality of one's sexuality—that is, whether it was of the ordinary variety or tantric in nature—was determined primarily by a person's ability to merge with the Self, enhanced by a meditative discipline, and, secondarily, by one's skill at going beyond the Self into radical union with another. The practice of tantra was likened to tending the flames of an inner sun which blazes forth from the sacred energy centers of the body, burning out negativity and purifying one's psyche. One is taken on an ecstatic, spiraling pilgrimage of sorts, from the base of the spine to the crown of the head and beyond. In the process, one discovers the supreme Self hidden deep within the heart. Union within and without awakens one to the inner shrine of cosmic and earthly love. Ultimately, this ancient art is capable of moving humanity beyond gender division and into alignment with the eternal Beloved Self.

Healing

In yoga, it is recognized that there are three levels of energy: tamas, raja, and satva. The first, tamas, relates to primal sexuality. With this level, one's sensitivity is underdeveloped. The next, raja, relates to unenlightened passions, such as deluded romantic and sexual behavior which is not grounded or aligned within the heart and body of Love—for example, promiscuity or adultery. Finally, satvic sexuality, which is the tantric or sacred path, incorporates beauty, meditative healing, heart-felt compassion, and mystical attunement, and is spiritually beneficial.

The appearance of the Calla Lily indicates that a major awakening is now available to your consciousness regarding sexuality and inner Love. The exotic birds, representing spiritual Love, and the two Calla Lilies, representing unity and balance, surround the Calla Lily cave where Beloved male and female consorts join in cosmic embrace. These tantric lovers wear orange tunics, the color of the second, sacral chakra, for they have found the ultimate creative expression which anchors and integrates this creative center within the human body. The color orange resonates with the vibrant hues of the rising sun, which when fully risen, radiates an awakened brilliance that burns away the ego. The lovers are gently held by the white Calla Lily, representing a kind of egoless cave of the heart, where two can truly meet and become One. Whether an individual pursuit or in relation to one's Beloved, the time has come to merge with these divine principles.

Practical Application

In my lectures on astrological cycles over the past three years I have emphasized a new potential coming into mass consciousness concerning our sexual and spiritual relationships. I have been predicting that many books and articles would soon become available on the topic of Tantric practices and Soul-centered sexuality, and this has come to pass.

If we wish, we are poised at this time in human evolution to become conscious of the healing aspects of sexuality as well as to open relationships to deeper areas of sacredness and trust. The Calla Lily essence can be most helpful in bringing this new, yet also very ancient, understanding of sacred sexuality into awareness and eventually into common practice. For this reason, I have included the Calla Lily in the Power of Flower deck. I am in the process of gathering stories and reports on how Calla Lily is assisting relationships at this time. Many of my women clients buy their husbands or partners astrological sessions as a gift. This will often lead to a joint session, where we examine the Soul patterns and dynamics between the two people in question, and, of course, sexuality is often a key area of concern. For example, how can the sexual union be preserved as sacred throughout a long term relationship? How can the couple access ever deeper intimacy and trust? And, in what ways can they work together to ensure health and vitality through sexual practice? Calla Lily is one of the best essences to offer these conscious couples. I recommend that it be taken together, at night, so that it may invoke the dream life and overlight the couple as they sleep and dream together. I have also recommended that it be used topically on the heart chakra and other intimate areas of the body, perhaps putting some in a favorite massage oil. I have mixed blends of Calla Lily, Rose, and Basil for couples who are pursuing sexual healing and Tantric mastery. I anticipate new stories and case histories will follow. Thus far, I have received many resounding affirmations that the essences are helping to balance and restore love to intimate relations.

Zinnia

LATIN: Zinnia elegans

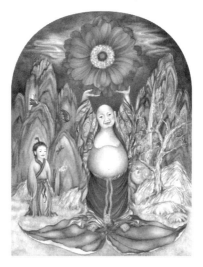

Blessing
Laughing Buddha, radiant one,
Carrying within the eternal Sun.
Shower your happiness on everyone.
Zinnia flowers so enchanting and bright,
My inner contentment shines with delight.

Plant Signature
*T*his summer annual is a glorious gift to any garden. The plant itself ranges in height from one to three feet, while its flower grows from one to five inches. It is called a double flower, due to its double row of petals which give the blossom an unusually full appearance. Colors include orange, rose, red, yellow, white, pink, and lavender.

Flower Essence

It is not surprising that people from all over the world gather to view zinnias in exhibitions and shows, for with their brilliant rainbow array of colors and abundance of petals, they are a luscious sight to behold, bringing much pleasure to the human heart. The flower essence derived from the zinnia is a treasure among nature's elixirs, for it enhances one's ability to rediscover the child-like qualities of playfulness, joy, delight, unconditional love, and a spirit of lighthearted innocence and adventure. Members of the fairy world, who are very child-like, themselves, take a special delight in the human cultivation of such qualities. This essence is highly recommended for anyone interested in reawakening their inner joy, as well as in countering lethargy and boredom. For example, it has an enlivening effect upon the elderly, and even animals (in particular, cats and dogs, have been known to become quite frisky under its influence). It is also recommended for people who work with children, for it attunes them to the wonders of the Child Mind.

Archetype
LAUGHING BUDDHA, PU-TAI

According to Chinese legend, the Buddha Pu-tai, also known as the Laughing Buddha, was an historical figure, a Chan (Zen) master, who lived sometime between the 6th and 10th centuries, and managed to discover the "Buddha within himself". He embodied perfect contentment, serenity, and happiness, and was often seen in the company of children, for whom he had a special fondness. After his death, he was elevated to the level of beloved cultural hero, and worshipped for his ability to bestow blessings of good fortune.

A jovial figure with round belly and protruding breasts, reminiscent of pre-Buddhist fertility goddesses from which he is in part derived, the Laughing Buddha radiates a quality of nurturing abundance to all who behold him. Though not officially recognized as a member of the pantheon of transcendent Buddhas, the Laughing Buddha is well known and loved as a protector of children by the common people of China and Japan. He lives on within the core of humanity as a bearer of Unconditional Love.

Healing

The Laughing Buddha holds aloft a bright orange zinnia—a great sphere of light or radiant Sun, showering its rays of happiness upon you. You are blessed beyond measure, for the Zinnia Laughing Buddha has come to celebrate the mirthful laughter of your joyous heart. What greater healing can come to you today than this?!

Po'Tai's robe is adorned with frolicking dolphins, the playful angels of the sea, whose very presence stirs the soul to its original innocence, bringing the essence of joy to the planet. The child at his side is in wonderment as a dragon-fly offers its gift of enchantment and beauty. These magical symbols are mirrors to your own divine gaiety. Breathe in the peace and contentment of the Laughing Buddha and discover within your own heart the many blessings he now brings to you.

Practical Application

The first time I used Zinnia was with my cat. As I was reviewing my essences one day, looking to see what I needed to reorder, the Zinnia essence seemed to jump out at me. I hadn't yet developed a close relationship with this particular essence, so I decided to go ahead, follow my impulse and pick it up. As I sat with the Zinnia, I received an inner picture of my cat, and I realized this was an essence for her. She had been very lethargic and depressed, and although not a playful cat by nature, seemed even more serious than usual. I made up an essence for Kitty Cake and witnessed a profound shift in her mood. The next day she displayed kitten-like qualities and was pawing at every dangling thing imaginable, even bumping into my legs more than usual as if to say, "Hey, let's play."

I am a person, who, by nature, does not enjoy being forced into situations where I'm expected to have fun. So for this reason, I have shied away from parties and fairs. In an attempt to lighten up, I decided to go to the Oregon Country Fair one year. Nudging myself out of resistance, I remembered Kitty Cake and her remarkable turn about with the Zinnia essence, so I gave it a try. Needless to say, I had lots of fun dancing to the fantastic music, and for the first time in many years, I just played. As a result, I decided to pay more attention to Zinnia, exploring ways I might use this essence to help others break through their inertia and melancholy.

The Laughing Buddha seemed a perfect archetype for Zinnia. The more I learned about Zinnia, the more I began to suspect that enlightenment was fundamentally about "lightening up." Have you ever noticed how light-hearted and playful the Dalai Lama is? So, I have learned, with the help of Zinnia, that play is just as virtuous as work. The Zinnia essence helps us recognize the abundance of joy that is available each and every day.

Zinnia helps us see life as one giant theatrical production. If we take ourselves and our stories too seriously, if we forget that we are actors in the Great Cosmic Play, or should I say the Great Cosmic Playground, we literally lose our sense of play. With Zinnia's help, we begin to see how truly comical things are. We start to giggle and pretty soon we are laughing and holding our sides, trying to catch our breath, and, finally, we are rolling around on the ground, weeping with gratitude because suddenly everything is just so darn funny. When we engage with our every day life in this manner, we come closer to actualizing the Laughing Buddha within ourselves. We do the dance of Lila, Divine Play.

Fuchsia

LATIN: Fuchsia hybrida

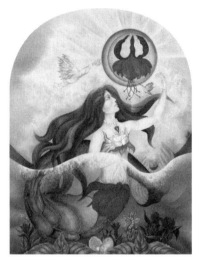

Blessing
Glory to Fuchsia,
For my suffering and pain,
And childhood past,
Are cleansed and soothed,
And healed at last.

Plant Signature

The fuchsia is a thick shrub with smooth green leaves. Its buds form in clusters, pointing toward the earth. Upon flowering in hues of red, pink and purple, its petals open upwards, crowning toward the heavens.

Flower Essence

As an elixir, this flower assists in the loving acceptance of long repressed core emotions—whether from this or other lifetimes. The special healing properties of the fuchsia guide one gently into deep, underwater caverns of the psyche, there to finally embrace one's long submerged and neglected grief, pain, and suffering. Often, through this process, the buried treasure of one's Real Self, whom we might call the Divine Child within, is revealed. By casting light into the emotional realms long held in darkness, fuchsia seeks to uplift the soul, elevating it to new levels of consciousness. Dark and light forces are reintegrated; one's vitality is enhanced.

Archetype
MERMAID

Known as "The Virgin of the Sea" or "Fish Tailed Aphrodite," the mermaid inhabits two worlds simultaneously: water (the emotions) and air (the intellect). On the one hand, her ability to descend to the depths of the sea gives her access to the hidden treasure of her Real Self. There, she overlights the dream world, for the deep sea is permeated with moon forces. On the other hand, her ability to ascend beyond the surface of the ocean waves, toward the sun and stars above, awakens her to higher levels consciousness. Around her neck are pearls of wisdom, salvaged from the buried treasure of her past. These she brings joyfully into the light of her future, the New World emerging within.

Healing

You must now learn to move freely between the watery realm of emotions and the arid world of the intellect. You are asked to courageously embrace life in all its dimensions, including pain and suffering, for in so doing, you strengthen yourself, allowing the spirit to travel beyond the confused emotions and perceptions of your personal history into the world of enchantment and true insight.

Ultimately, like the fish-tailed Goddess, you emerge into wholeness; that which was once only known in the dark, womb-like places, is now fully integrated in the light of day.

When the Fuchsia mermaid visits you she invokes your long awaited transformation. The cherub angel pictured above her head represents your Divine Child, freed from the confines of the past and now heralding your glorious rebirth. Joyously, the hummingbird overlights you, for you have found many treasures buried in the darkness of your suffering and now know yourself to be whole in the midst of all that life has to offer. Rise up and receive the many blessings of your New World.

Practical Application

Fuchsia has always been a favorite flower of mine. There were Fuchsia plants growing all around our house in northern California when I was a little girl. My sister and I would run around the yard popping the Fuchsia bulbs open and delighting in the happy clusters of open flowers that resembled fairies hanging from the vine. So, as an adult, when I learned that Fuchsia essence was used to heal childhood trauma and bring the unconscious aspects of our Soul Self into conscious light, I was deeply moved. I have no doubt that the plant was a protector for me as a child, and when I have used the essence, I feel a deep kinship with its healing properties.

There are certain flowers that may have played an important role in your life at different times. Often, these flowers come up for clients in their sessions, and it is like a sweet friend from the past knocking upon the door of one's Soul. My stepfather was a quiet man whom I respected and loved very much, though there was little overt display of our mutual appreciation for each other. However, every year in the month of May, on my birthday, he would purchase a flat of pansies that we would plant in the front of the house. I remember skipping around the house, heralding the Fuchsia, draping the shady side of the house, and the bright pansy faces peering up at the sun, from the sunny side of the house, on warm Summer afternoons. My love for these two flowers make them an excellent remedy combination for my own childhood issues.

I believe our wounded nature is the unpolished jewel of precious qualities and gifts that becomes our highest gift to the world when uncovered and polished with the work of our conscious desire to heal and serve. Fuchsia elixir offers us the ability to move freely between the watery realms of the past and the spirit-filled heavens of conscious intent.

The Fuchsia essence is often prescribed for children and adults who have been sexually abused; those who carry the burden of this trauma deep in the treasure chest of the past. Fuchsia holds the key that unlocks the past, and so is very useful in this kind of Inner Child work, in particular. Combined with the guidance of a trained professional, the remedy is especially potent, gently but firmly helping one open to painful memories and, in general, assisting in the healing process. It also works very well for therapists who do past-life recall work and hypnotherapy. A beautiful floral essence combination is Fuchsia, Golden Ear Drops, Bleeding Heart, and Pomegranate. Black-Eyed Susan can be taken as well, but its effects stimulate a deeper access to pain, and may be a bit much for some people, especially children.

Angel's Trumpet

LATIN: Datura candida

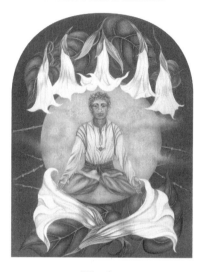

Blessing
Angel's Trumpet,
Sound a note,
New World Man, Arise!
Heal the wounded male within,
Make him whole, Make him wise.

Plant Signature

*A*lso known as Brugmansia, this large evergreen shrub can be trained as a small tree. With ample leaves and flowers, Angel's Trumpet can be somewhat dominating in the garden. Especially fragrant at night, its shiny, tubular flowers point downward toward the earth, closely resembling trumpets, shimmering beautifully in the moonlight.

Flower Essence

Often times, we fear change. For even in its most positive form, something that is familiar must die so that something as yet unknown can be born in its place. At the threshold of life's many transitions, a leap of faith is required, and with this leap, it becomes clear that one is no longer in control of external circumstances. The illusion of certainty is shattered, and one is invited to acknowledge and make peace with the fundamental uncertainty of earthly existence—with the fact that everything that is born must eventually die.

In the face of life's inevitable changes, Angel's Trumpet offers its trumpet-like call, heralding a time of transformation and rebirth, while ushering in the highest awareness of spiritual assistance and loosening the grip of ego identification, so that a pure heart and mind can be gracefully realized and set free. Angel's Trumpet is especially helpful for those who resist letting go of material attachments, for it teaches the important lesson that surrender into spirit is the only way to true peace and freedom. Similarly, the elixir can assist those who are engaged in a literal dying process, as well as those who are transitioning from one state of consciousness to another. Ultimately, this succulent blossom trumpets the song of the human soul, releasing one from the path of suffering through an opening to the ineffable beauty of life.

Archetype
New World Man

A great tragedy has occurred over the course of the last 5,000 years of human history, stemming from a profound imbalance between the masculine and feminine principles which have prevailed down through the millennia. Violations to nature and women, as well as to alternative medical and political systems, are but a few of the areas where male-domination has caused great harm to the planet. Much healing must occur within the male archetype and humanity must realize that the dominant paradigms of the past have been misguided and unskillful. Such a realization would, in no way, diminish man's co-creative partnership with the Divine in establishing a true Paradise on Earth.

Angel's Trumpet flowers humbly bow toward the earth, sounding a note of reverence to Her sustenance and wisdom. It is through a deep surrender of the personal will to control and dominate, that the New World Man will become capable of healthy expressions of creativity and assertion, and fulfill his considerable destiny of service to humanity.

New World Man is undergoing a great transformation at this time on the planet. His core understanding of what it means to be male is in the process of being completely revamped, in order that he may become balanced in heart and mind, deepen his attunement with his own internal God Man, and find non-reactive solutions to the problem of survival in a world of limited resources and human imperfection. For women, the relationship to our own inner male is in serious need of compassionate repair, as well.

Everything must change. The form of the Old World does not sustain the evolving consciousness emanating from the hearts of humanity at this time. In order to reclaim his essential beauty and goodness, man must cultivate the virtue of self-sacrifice. Radical and skillful means must be embraced in order to finally and fully surrender into the field of pure, enlightened consciousness—the only place from which the New World Man can meet the challenges of worldly existence and planetary custodianship without splintering into wounded distortions of his True Male Self.

New World Man is reuniting with kindred spirits and universal truths as he weaves his way back into the web of interconnectedness which supports ecological well-being, political justice, racial freedom, women's empowerment, and cultural diversity. His receptivity to change happens only when he understands that he must be transformed internally, so that he may blossom in aspiration with the Divine.

Healing

For both men and women, Angel's Trumpet beckons you to surrender inwardly, to the areas in your life that are in need of repair, compassion, and re-ordering at this time. This card comes to remind you that in the correct ordering of things, outer manifestation should come only as a crowning of the inner being, after one has truly opened to joy and a willingness to change. If you are inwardly receptive at this time, you will receive the subtle insights and messages necessary for integration and wholeness.

Angel's Trumpet flowers shine in the evening—the white blossoms glowing under the illumined moon. Symbolically, it is vital for New World Man, and the male principle in each woman, to enter his garden in the evening hours, allowing the receptive moon to stir his soul. Flowers are very receptive, and they will delight in being asked to participate in the healing of male woundedness. New World Man embraces nature, and by association, woman, in all Her integrity. He humbly walks a path toward the future in order that he may help build a New World—a world of justice, harmony, and balance.

Practical Application

Angel's Trumpet is often used during major transitions in a person's life when crossing a threshold into a new dimension of consciousness, whether through actual death or powerful surrender to the unknown. Indeed, I have seen this essence work wonders.

My mother's death was a profound experience for my sister and myself as we learned how to care for her during her last month of life, and were given the honor of watching over her as she died at peace in her own home. A strong woman all of her life, my mother clung to life until the very end. When it was her time to surrender out of her physical body, she exhibited some anxiety and tension. We administered Angel's Trumpet essence under her tongue along with

Rose and Aspen. Her face changed dramatically within ten minutes. It appeared as if all of the wrinkles of time had disappeared. My mother died soon afterwards, with an angel's smile. We bathed her body in Rose water and dressed her in fresh pink pajamas. I placed a crystal and a Rose on her chest, and let her lie in peace for some time. Later, when her friends came to say one last goodbye, they all commented on how beautiful and young she looked. My mother, with the help of the flower angels, left this world with grace.

My reason for connecting Angel's Trumpet to the archetype of New World Man is because we as a culture must die to the old world structures and patriarchal paradigms, while embracing feminine wisdom and insights. For this to happen, the men of the world, in particular, have some deep and sustained work with the Will ahead of them. The necessary surrender toward new modalities of masculine expression will call for profound shifts in the mass consciousness of Man.

I currently have two male clients who have been experimenting with Angel's Trumpet, visualizing the potential of New World Man as they take their daily doses. They have reported some internal shifts of consciousness. The most significant has been with regard to their primary relationships, where each has found more of a willingness to let go of old ways and habits, and to truly listen to the needs of their partners.

Once becoming acquainted with the power of flower essences, you can't help but become a flower messenger. Upon hearing of a friend's illness or crisis, the first thing that comes to mind is "They need flowers!" I often hear the call of Angel's Trumpet at such times.

Morning Glory

LATIN: Ipomoea purpurea

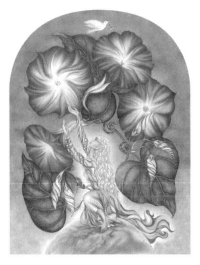

Blessing
Morning Glory,
The Goddess anew,
A flowering vine,
In radiant blue.
I speak my truth, I live my dreams,
I am vibrant, alive, and fully seen.

Plant Signature

A summer annual plant, the Morning Glory is beautifully adorned with large, bell-like flowers, their smooth, funnel-shaped throats widening out around the edges. Nestled among heart-shaped leaves, these blossoms—typically a radiant blue, though colors may vary—connect at the top of each bell to a twisting stem which can be found climbing along fence posts and rock walls. Most Morning Glories open only in the morning, positioning their blossomy heads upward.

Flower Essence

The glorious spectacle of this beautiful plant as it blooms in the early morning sun, awakens one to the essential harmonies of nature, and inspires a renewed sense of soulful enthusiasm. Likewise, as a flower elixir, Morning Glory awakens the spirit, attuning the individual to his or her own shimmering brilliance and vitality. It can serve as a rejuvenating tonic, melting away patterns of lethargy or inertia. The essence allows one to feel embraced by the jubilant forces of nature, and ushers in a "Newly Awakened Self."

Archetype
NEW WORLD GODDESS

Spiritual beauty is the ultimate truth which permeates and enchants the world. All the glitter and glamour of our modern culture cannot compare to the natural radiance of the individual who awakens to spirit. For through this enlightening transformation we create love, embody love, and realize love—manifesting the greatest beauty and power to be found on Earth. In other words, we become the New World Goddess.

Just as Morning Glory blossoms glow and sparkle in the shimmering radiance of the glorious rising sun, each cell of the New World Goddess' body becomes luminous upon awakening to the Light. And just as the Morning Glory is adorned with heart-shaped leaves, so the New World Goddess is adorned with loving images and symbols. With grace and splendor, She remembers her Self to be awake. An ardent prayer of gratitude rises in her heart, for she is again, and always has been, one with Anima Mundi, the World Soul. Her body dances like a divine instrument, while musical notes symbolize the truth that

She sings and speaks. Fully realized in every woman and man, the New World Goddess spontaneously and effortlessly offers Her beauty to the Supreme. She is awakened in all Her sacred, feminine glory.

Healing

Whether you are male or female, this card is a fervent call to the realization of your own unique destiny, as well as to the future evolution of humanity. Just as nature aspires to perfect itself for the ultimate benefit of All, so too, humanity seeks perfection as its most sublime offering and final destination. The time has come for you to truly embrace the New World Goddess—the sacred, feminine center which brings the beauty of perfection to all actions, deeds, and creations. Seek resolution; let the Old World die away; listen to the new voice emerging within your mind and heart. There can be no more lies, curses, or harmful conduct. Heeding the call of the Millennial Oracle, the New World Woman now at last reemerges from the sleeping womb of the last five thousand years. You awaken with Her—alive, vibrant, and renewed. Speak and affirm the Supreme perfection that you are.

Practical Application

You might wonder why I have associated Morning Glory with the New World Goddess, since this particular essence is indicated when a person is feeling numb, dull, drained, unable to rest deeply—in short, world weary. Precisely! This is the condition in which many of us find ourselves as we attempt to "have it all," according to an outmoded, masculine model of success. It seems we got both less and more than we bargained for—less unstructured, quality time with ourselves and our loved ones; and more stress-related health problems like chronic fatigue syndrome, insomnia, heart disease, high blood pressure, lung cancer, infertility and depression.

A women in need of Morning Glory often says that she

doesn't want to get up in the morning and face another day. I have recommended Morning Glory essence to many women who are lacking in life force due to the fierce demands of an overburdened life. Blessedly, this essence puts a woman in touch with the real source of vitality and the rhythms of Nature, so that she may begin to reinvent the role of the feminine in healthier and more fulfilling ways. It takes courage and discipline, oddly enough, to slow down and ask ourselves what our real needs are. When we address these real needs, we begin to have more respect for life, and for our unfolding destiny as women on the planet. Perhaps at your next women's circle, you can all make a toast to Morning Glory, and imagine together what a New World Goddess looks, acts and feels like. Please join me in doing this.

For men, Morning Glory essence can awaken a fresh perspective, as well, and when attuning to the New World Goddess, men are invited to explore new understanding and ways of relating to the their own feminine sides.

Alchemy

The Flowering of the New World Soul

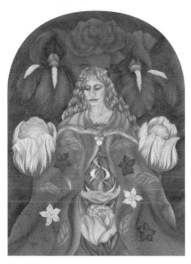

*A*lchemy is a powerful blend of exoteric (scientific) and esoteric (mystical) wisdom which seeks to illuminate the ultimate secrets of Nature as well as the soul development of humanity. This Wild Card of the Power of Flowers deck includes all of the potentials held within the individual cards. With its appearance, you are given the privilege of sorting through the remaining cards in the deck in order to choose for yourself the flower and archetype which best assist you now on your alchemical journey toward Self-Realization.

The Alchemy card holds a special message for you, for pictured here is Natura, The Goddess of Nature, cloaked in Her garment of Nature's Angels, the many flowers of Her world. Situated between the sun and the moon—Sol and Luna, the cosmic opposites—Natura is crowned with the stars of the heavens. She stands upon a crescent moon, representing Her moist and fertile mysteries. Spiraling within Her womb, New World Soul gestates, receiving its encoded DNA cell structure from Her bank of Universal Wisdom. This new being of light, who might be called "Cosmic Consciousness," represents the evolutionary future of humanity—where one is in sync with both temporal and heavenly attributes: As Above, So Below. With this card comes a text known as "The Emerald Tablet," which you are asked to read aloud. Contemplate these words and know them for the eternal truth they represent—a wisdom passed down through the ages in order that we may come to realize that which we already are—a Flowering New World Soul.

The Emerald Tablet

1. True, without deceit, certain and most true.

2. What is below, is like what is above, and what is above is like that which is below, for the performing of the marvels of the One.

3. And as all things proceed from the One, through the meditation of the One; so all things proceed from this one thing, by adaptation.

4. Its father is the sun, its mother is the moon; the wind hath carried it in its belly; its nurse is the earth.

5. This is the father of all perfection of the whole world.

6. Its power is complete when it is turned towards the earth.

7. You shall separate the earth from the fire, the subtle from the gross, smoothly and with great cleverness.

8. It ascends from the earth to heaven, and descends again to the earth, and receives the power of the higher and the lower things. So shall you have the glory of the whole world. So shall all the obscurity yield before thee.

9. This is the strong fortitude of all fortitude: because it will overcome every subtle thing and penetrate every solid.

10. Thus was the world created.

11. Hence will there be marvelous adaptations, of which this is the means.

12. And so I am called Hermes Trismegistus, as having three parts of the philosophy of the whole world.

13. What I have said concerning the operation of the sun is finished.

Tabula Smaragdina or The Emerald Tablets of Hermes, the Magna Carta of Alchemy

Epilogue

Flowers are the moment's representations of things that are in themselves eternal.

— Sri Aurobindo

Life must blossom like a flower offering itself to the Divine.

— The Mother

Historically, as one civilization evolves into the next, an urgent and familiar call for transformation and rebirth can be heard. Prophetic teachings, predicting the course of humanity's evolutionary trajectory, have existed everywhere on the globe throughout history. As we trace such divinely inspired pronouncements, we will surely recognize a consistent theme of unrelenting hunger for ultimate reunion with the Divine essence of our Soul, and along with this long-awaited reunion, an answer to life's great mysteries.

As we approach the twenty-first century, we find ourselves at a crucial turn of the evolutionary spiral, for we stand poised on the brink of destroying Mother Earth—our precious home. Humanity's co-creative work with the natural world has diminished sharply over the last several centuries, causing severe damage to the fragile eco-system upon which we rely for our continued existence. Never before has the necessity of balancing material and spiritual realities been so urgently apparent. For without such a balancing, we will surely not survive. We must spiritualize our priorities as a global community, and if nothing else, seek to merge our hearts and minds with the Soul of Nature. Given the vast array of religious beliefs which inevitably divide us, it is imperative that we look to the trees, flowers, oceans, mountains, and plants for the universalizing wisdom we so clearly lack. Nature holds the secrets of the universe in its abundant embrace—speaking a language which transcends our many differences, while anchoring the Divine in material form.

The Age of Flowers is upon us. Let us receive, with utmost humility, the many blessings of these gentle beings. Let us also remember that the movement toward perfection is not limited to the human realm. Indeed, it is through the perfection of Nature and Her sublime rhythms that we come to embrace the passage of time, and surrender to the many transformations in our lives, in harmony and unconditional gratitude. In the words of Sri Aurobindo:

> *Lo! Here are flowers and benedictions!*
> *Here is the smile of divine Love!*
> *It is without preferences and without repulsions.*
> *It streams out toward all in a generous flow and*
> *never takes back its marvelous gifts!*

The more we unite with Nature, the more we experience its healing balm of compassion. The flower beings overflow with tenderness and love for humanity, and they long to merge with us—to share a common field of experience and sympathy. They assist and inspire us in so many ways—through flower essence energy, fragrance, color, and beauty. All of nature rejoices at the crowning glory of the floral world.

As the final words of this book are written, I, its author, am in awe of the spiritual wisdom of Nature and the many gifts She bestows upon us if we will only open our hearts to Her beauty. With much gratitude in my heart for Her countless blessings, I invite you to surrender to Nature's call as you walk your path lightly upon the Earth. Like the flowers that grace our planet, let us live each day anew.

— Isha Lerner

Flower Essence Companies

Alaskan Flower Essence Project
P.O. Box 1369
Homer, AK 99603-1369

Desert Alchemy
P.O. Box 44189
Tucson, AZ 85733

Findhorn Flower Essences
"Wellspring"
31 The Park
Findhorn Bay
Moray, Scotland
IV36 3TY

www.Pacific Essences .Com
P.O. Box 8317 384-5560
Victoria, BC V8W 3R9
Canada

Flower Essences Services
P.O. Box 1769
Nevada City, CA 95959

Bibliography

Cunningham, Donna, *Flower Remedies Handbook: Emotional Healing and Growth with Bach and Other Flower Essences.* New York, NY: Sterling Publishing Co., Inc., 1992.

Fabricius, Johannes, *Alchemy: The Medieval Alchemists and their Royal Art.* Rev. ed. London: Diamond Books, 1989.

Fischer-Rizzi, Suzanne, *Complete Aromatherapy Handbook: Essential Oils for Radiant Health.* Trans. and Ed. Elisabeth E. Hartman and Jeanette Green. New York, NY: Sterling Publishing Co., Inc., 1990.

Howard, Judy and John Ramsell, Curators and Trustees. *The Original Writings of Edward Bach: Compiled from the Archives of the Dr. Edward Bach Healing Trust,* Mount Vernon, Sotwel, Essex: The C.W. Daniel Company Limited, 1990.

Kaminski, Patricia and Richard Katz, *Flower Essence Repertory: A Comprehensive Selection Guide for the Natural Health Practitioner.* Rev. and exp. Nevada City: The Flower Essence Society, 1992.

Reader's Digest, *Magic and Medicine of Plants: A Practical Guide to the Science, History, Folklore, and Everyday Uses of Medicinal Plants.* Pleasantville, NY, Montreal: The Reader's Digest Association, Inc., 1986.

von Franz, Marie-Louise, *Alchemy: An Introduction to the Symbolism and the Psychology.* Toronto: Inner City Books, 1980.

About the Author

Isha Lerner has been an international astrologer, tarot consultant, and flower essence practitioner for over twenty years. She spent four years living at the Findhorn Foundation in Scotland in the 1970s studying and experiencing the co-creative relationship between humanity, nature, and mysticism. She co-authored the Inner Child Cards: A Journey Through Fairy Tales, Myth, and Nature in 1993, and her latest publication, The Power of Flowers Cards: An Archetypal Journey Through Nature is an extension of her continued study of plant lore, flower essence therapy, mythology, and archetype. Isha has a thriving practice in Eugene, Oregon where she resides with her three daughters. She is available for long-distance consultations, workshops, and lectures.

To contact Isha:

Isha Lerner
P.O. BOX 5164
Eugene, OR 97405
isha@efn.org
www. ishalerner.com

Also by Isha Lerner:

The Inner Child Cards:
A Journey Through Fairy Tales, Myth, and Nature

Books by Donna Cunningham:

Flower Remedies Handbook:
Emotional Healing and Growth With Bach
and Other Flower Essences

How To Read Your Astrological Chart:
Aspects of the Cosmic Puzzle